Nephrology pocket

MW01006632

Authors:

Alexander S. Goldfarb-Rumyantzev, M.D., Ph.D
Nephrology Division
Beth Israel Deaconess Medical Center
Assistant Professor of Medicine
Harvard Medical School
Boston, MA 02215

Robert S. Brown, M.D.
Clinical Chief, Nephrology Division
Beth Israel Deaconess Medical Center
Associate Professor of Medicine
Harvard Medical School
Boston, MA 02215

© 2014, by Börm Bruckmeier Publishing, LLC
111 ½ Eucalyptus Drive
El Segundo, CA 90245
www.media4u.com | Ph: (310) 414 8300

Acknowledgments
The authors wish to acknowledge the editorial help of Dr. Sharyu Kailas Gangwal who made our charts, figures & algorithms look good & the late Dr. Richard Nesson & Iris International, Inc. IQ200 system for providing several urinary crystal photomicrographs. In addition, we recognize that our roles as teachers of clinical medicine & nephrology to students & young physicians at Harvard Medical School and the Beth Israel Deaconess Medical Center provided the inspiration to write this book directed toward learning about renal & electrolyte disorders.

Editing: Sharyu Gangwal, MD; Nathalie Blanck, MD; Dominik Stauber, MD
Production: Anne Herhold, Alexander Storck, Rohit Kumar, Deepak Sahu
Cover image: fotolia.com

IMPORTANT NOTICE – PLEASE READ!
This book is based on information from sources believed to be reliable, and every effort has been made to make the book as complete and accurate as possible and to describe generally accepted practices based on information available as of the printing date, but its accuracy & completeness cannot be guaranteed. Despite the best efforts of author & publisher, the book may contain errors, and the reader should use the book only as a general guide & not as the ultimate source of information about the subject matter. This book is not intended to reprint all of the information available to the author or publisher on the subject, but rather to simplify, complement and supplement other available sources. The reader is encouraged to read all available material & to consult the package insert & other references to learn as much as possible about the subject. This book is sold without warranties of any kind, expressed or implied, & the publisher & author disclaim any liability, loss or damage caused by the content of this book.
IF YOU DO NOT WISH TO BE BOUND BY THE FOREGOING CAUTIONS AND CONDITION, YOU MAY RETURN THIS BOOK TO THE PUBLISHER FOR A FULL REFUND.

ISBN 978-1-59103-270-0
Printed in China through Colorcraft Ltd., Hong Kong

Preface

Nephrology, the subspecialty of internal medicine which covers the diagnosis and treatment of kidney diseases, hypertension, electrolyte and acid-base disorders, dialysis and kidney transplantation, is often viewed as very difficult to master. Moreover, the major textbooks available offer more information than general internists, family physicians, physician assistants, nurse practitioners, medical residents, fellows, and students usually require.

This **Nephrology Pocket** is structured to provide the essential data to evaluate, understand, and manage most of the commonly seen disorders in the clinical practice of nephrology and which should be known to general medical caregivers. The book is in a form that can be kept in your coat pocket or on an electronic reader that can be used on rounds or in clinic. The content of each of the 16 chapters is divided into subtopics in the Table of Contents that guide the reader directly to charts and algorithms providing pertinent information quickly. This format also allows us to keep the information up to date whenever new evidence becomes available.

We feel sure that you will find this a helpful reference that you want to keep with you in your daily practice. We welcome any criticism or suggestions from our readers as well. Please contact us at info@media.com

The authors and publisher   October 2013

Alexander S. Goldfarb-Rumyantzev, M.D., Ph.D
Robert S. Brown, M.D.

Dedication

To my Mom Tatiana, my uncle Vena and my children Levi and Ben – my constant source of inspiration.

Alexander S. Goldfarb-Rumyantzev, M.D., Ph.D

To the late Frank Epstein – mentor, colleague, and friend for 40 years.

Robert S. Brown, M.D.

4   Contents

6   Contents

8 Contents

10   Contents

1   Introduction to Nephrology

Nephrology, the subspecialty of internal medicine which covers the diagnosis and treatment of kidney diseases, hypertension, and electrolyte disorders, is often viewed as very difficult to master.

In this Nephrology Pocket book, we will break the field of renal and electrolyte disorders down into tables and algorithms that allow the reader a simplified, yet comprehensive, approach to nephrology. One can't become a nephrologist in a month, but the reader can master the major areas of the specialty to a surprising degree of sophistication in the course of a 4-week rotation.

Start with a brief review of Chapters 1–4:

> Chapter 1) Introduction,
> Chapter 2) Symptoms, Signs and Differential Diagnosis,
> Chapter 3) Renal Physiology, and
> Chapter 4) Urinalysis and Diagnostic Tests.

Then review the data in the remaining chapters specified for each week as follows:

Week 1: Chapter 5) Water and Electrolyte Disorders
Chapter 6) Acid-base Disorders

Week 2: Chapter 7) Glomerular Diseases
Chapter 8) Interstitial, Cystic, Obstructive, and Infectious Kidney Diseases
Chapter 9) Kidney Disorders in Other Diseases

Week 3: Chapter 10) Hypertension and Renal Artery Stenosis
Chapter 11) Kidney Stones
Chapter 12) Acute Kidney Injury/Acute Renal Failure

Week 4: Chapter 13) Chronic Kidney Diseases
Chapter 14) Dialysis
Chapter 15) Kidney Transplantation

This presupposes that the reader already has a basic knowledge of renal patho-physiology and function, body fluids, and metabolic disorders as taught in the second year of medical school, but a review of the Renal Physiology chapter will be a helpful memory refresher.

Let us first review the patient issues that will be the subject of most nephrology referrals or consultations.

1.1　Common Nephrology Consultations

Condition	Look For	
• Acute kidney injury (AKI) or acute renal failure (ARF) • Etiology - prerenal, postrenal, intrinsic renal disease	• Creatinine (Cr) increase with daily trend • History and physical examination (Hx & Px) for edema/volume depletion	• Urinalysis (UA) • Serum electrolytes, calcium, phosphate • Urine chemistries (Cr, Na, Osm) • Renal ultrasound (US) • Urine output (UO)
• Chronic kidney disease (CKD) or chronic renal failure. • Etiology of nephrotic syndrome, nephritis, or systemic diseases involving the kidneys	• Cr increase with weekly or monthly trend, • Hx & Px for edema/volume depletion • Urinalysis • Urine output • Renal US	• Anemia • Cholesterol • Albumin • Ca^{2+}/phos/bone disorders • Acidosis • Parathyroid hormone (PTH)
• Evaluation of electrolyte disorders & volume status • Hypo/hypernatremia, hypo/hyperkalemia	• Hx & Px for edema/volume depletion • Creatinine • Urine output	• Urine "electrolytes" (U_{Na^+}, U_{K^+}, U_{Cl^-}) • U_{Cr}, U_{Osm}
• Calcium, phosphate &/or magnesium disorders	• Hyper/hypocalcemia • Hyper/hypophosphatemia • Hyper/hypoparathyroidism	• Vitamin D levels • Bone pathology
• Nephrolithiasis, management and prevention	• Need for urologic intervention • Stone composition • Crystalluria	• Blood tests • 24 hr urine chemistries for supersaturation
• Need for hemodialysis (HD), peritoneal dialysis (PD), continuous renal replacement therapy (CRRT), vascular access or options counseling in end-stage renal disease (ESRD) or acute renal failure (ARF) patients	• Uremic symptoms • Volume overload/CHF • Uncontrollable hyperkalemia or acidosis • Low creatinine clearance • Pericarditis	• Encephalopathy • Uremic coagulopathy

Condition (cont.)	Look For	
• Hypertension, controlled, uncontrolled, accelerated or malignant	• Evaluate for secondary causes vs "essential" and for end-organ damage	• Management with specific drug indications
• Acid-base disorders	• Arterial or venous pH • HCO_3 • pCO_2	• Anion gap • Serum electrolytes
• Adjustment of medications in renal disease or transplant patients	• Renal vs hepatic excretion	• Knowledge of immunosuppressive drugs

1.2 Follow-up Assessments of Nephrology Patients

- Etiology of renal disease based on test results
- Kidney function & trend
- Volume status, input and output (I&O)
- Electrolytes and acid-base status
- Hypertension (HTN)
- Anemia
- Calcium balance, hyperphosphatemia, hyperparathyroidism, bone disorders
- Appropriate doses of medications with renal excretion
- Systemic disease status, if present
- Need for dialysis, vascular access & dialysis adequacy or kidney transplantation
- Nutritional status & hypoalbuminemia
- Concomitant conditions: cardiac, respiratory, infectious, gastrointestinal, neurologic diseases

1.3 General Overview of Renal Diseases

Glomerular
Nephritic syndromes

• Acute post-infectious glomerulonephritis (immune complex deposition)
• Rapidly progressive GN - crescentic GN
  - Immune complex deposition (eg, endocarditis)
  - Antibody deposition (eg, Goodpasture's syndrome)
  - Pauci-immune (eg, ANCA positive, granulomatosis with polyangitis (formerly Wegener's granulomatosis))
• Membrano-proliferative GN (immune complex deposition, eg, hepatitis C, SLE)
• Mesangial proliferative GN (immune complex deposition, eg, IgA nephropathy, SLE)

Glomerular (cont.)

Nephrotic syndromes

- Minimal change disease (lipoid nephrosis)
- Membranous nephropathy (immune complex deposition)
- Focal segmental glomerular sclerosis
- Collapsing glomerulopathy
- Secondary nephrotic syndrome (diabetes, tumors, HIV, amyloidosis, malaria, syphilis, drugs)

Vascular

- Benign/malignant hypertensive nephrosclerosis
- Renal artery stenosis (arteriosclerosis, fibromuscular dysplasia)
- Renal artery occlusion (thrombosis, emboli)
- Renal arteriolar disease (HUS/TTP thrombotic microangiopathy, preeclampsia, atherosclerosis)
- Vasculitis (polyarteritis nodosa, cryoglobulinemia, scleroderma)
- Bilateral renal vein thrombosis

Interstitial

- Chronic pyelonephritis and other kidney infections.
- Allergic interstitial nephritis (usually drug-induced)
- Analgesic nephropathy
- Papillary necrosis
- Sarcoid nephritis, Sjögren syndrome
- Tubulointerstitial nephritis with iritis

Tubular

- Ischemic or nephrotoxic ATN
- Myoglobinuria, hemoglobinuria
- Hypercalcemic nephropathy, milk-alkali syndrome
- Crystal deposition - Urate nephropathy, oxalosis, phosphate nephropathy
- Toxic nephropathies (lithium, heavy metals, "herbal" aristolochic acid nephropathy)

Others

- Polycystic kidneys
- Obstructive nephropathy
- Renal-cell carcinoma, other infiltrative diseases
- Renal stones
- Multiple myeloma (light chain or cast nephropathy, amyloidosis)
- Tuberous sclerosis, hereditary diseases

For additional data, see specific chapter headings in the table of contents.

2   Symptoms, Signs & Differential Diagnosis

2.1   Edema

2.1.1   Renal

Probable Diagnosis	Symptoms/Signs	Diagnostic Procedures
Nephrotic syndrome	• Facial swelling • Arms, legs swelling esp. ankles and feet • Pleural effusions • Foamy urination • Weight gain (water retention)	• Urine protein/creatinine ratio or 24 hr protein • Blood urea nitrogen (BUN) • Serum creatinine • Serum albumin • Creatinine clearance (CrCl) • Urinalysis (UA) • Renal biopsy
Nephritic syndrome eg, acute glomerulo-nephritis)	• Peripheral or periorbital edema • Hematuria • Oliguria • Headache - secondary to hypertension • Shortness of breath or dyspnea on exertion - secondary to heart failure • Possible flank pain secondary to stretching of the renal capsule	• UA and urinary sediment for protein, red blood cells (RBCs), white blood cells (WBCs), casts • Serum electrolytes, BUN, creatinine • Serologic tests for C3, C4, ASLO, ANCA, anti-GBM and hepatitis antibodies • Renal ultrasonography (USG) and renal biopsy
Chronic kidney disease (CKD)	• Swelling - generalized (fluid retention), ankle, foot, and leg • High blood pressure • Nausea or vomiting • Loss of appetite • Metallic taste in mouth • Flank pain • Hyperkalemia, metabolic acidosis • Urination changes: Oliguria, anuria, nocturia (excessive urination at night) • Fatigue	• Blood tests- Creatinine, BUN, electrolytes, CBC, calcium, phosphate, albumin. • Urine tests - CrCl, 24 hour urinary protein or urine protein to creatinine ratio • Arterial or venous blood gas, if serum bicarbonate is low. • Renal USG • Renal biopsy if indicated and kidneys are not contracted and small • Abdominal CT scan or MRI when indicated by USG findings

2.1.2   Cardiovascular

Probable Diagnosis	Symptoms/Signs	Diagnostic Procedures
Congestive heart failure (CHF)	• Swelling (edema) of the ankles and legs or abdomen. • Crackles • S_3 gallop • Dyspnea (shortness of breath) • Cough • Fatigue, weakness, faintness • Loss of appetite • Palpitations • Swollen (enlarged) liver or abdomen • Neck veins distended • Increased urination at night (nocturia) • Weight gain	• Electrocardiogram (ECG) • Echocardiogram (echo) • Chest X-ray • Angiography • Blood test-BNP (B-type natriuretic peptide) level
Cardiomyopathy	• Shortness of breath or trouble breathing, especially with physical exertion • Chest pain • Fatigue (tiredness) • Swelling in the ankles, feet, legs, abdomen, and veins in the neck • Dizziness, fainting • Lightheadedness • Arrhythmias (irregular heartbeats) • Heart murmurs	• Physical examination [Tachypnea, tachycardia, hypertension, hypoxia, jugular venous distension (JVD), pulmonary edema (crackles and/or wheezes), S3 gallop] • Plasma brain natriuretic peptide (BNP) • Chest X-ray, MRI • Heart catheterization

2.1.3 Endocrine

Probable Diagnosis	Symptoms/Signs	Diagnostic Procedures
Cushing's syndrome	• Round, red, full face (moon face) • Cervical fat pads • Comedones (acne) • Purplish pink stretch marks (striae) • Fatigue, headache, weak muscles, • High blood pressure, high blood sugars, hypokalemia • Polydipsia and polyuria • Loss of libido, depression	• Clinical evaluation • Serum and salivary cortisol level, ACTH levels • Dexamethasone suppression test • 24-hour urinary measurement for cortisol • Abdominal CT scanning of adrenal glands and MRI of pituitary gland • Bone density
Hypothyroidism	• Puffy face, hands, and swelling of the legs • Increased sensitivity to cold • Fatigue or feeling slowed down • Joint or muscle pain • Coarse hair or brittle fingernails • Dry skin • Muscle cramps	• Clinical evaluation • Thyroid function tests (TFT's) • Thyroid releasing hormone (TRH) test • MRI of the brain

2.1.4   Others

Probable Diagnosis	Symptoms/Signs	Diagnostic Procedures
Cirrhosis	• Swelling or fluid buildup of the legs (edema) and in the abdomen (ascites • Confusion or problems thinking • Loss of appetite • Nausea and vomiting • Nosebleeds or bleeding gums • Pale or clay-colored stools • Small, red spider-like blood vessels on the skin (spider angiomas) • Yellow color in the skin, mucus membranes, or eyes (jaundice) • Impotence, loss of libido	• CBC, liver function tests (LFTs) • CT or MRI of the abdomen • Endoscopy to check for abnormal variceal veins in the esophagus or stomach • Abdominal USG • A liver biopsy confirming cirrhosis • Levels of alpha fetoprotein (AFP)
Preeclampsia	• Swelling of face or legs • Severe headaches • Hypertension, hyper-reflexia • Blurry vision, flashing lights, and floaters • Vomiting and pain in the upper abdomen • A decrease in urine output	• CBC with differential and platelet count • Check for proteinuria • 24 hr urine collection for creatinine clearance and total protein • Fetal USG • LFTs

2.2 Hypertension

Probable Diagnosis	Symptoms/Signs	Diagnostic Procedures
CKD	(see 2.1.1 Renal) →15	
Hyperthyroidism	• High blood pressure • Difficulty concentrating • Fatigue • Frequent bowel movements • Goiter (visibly enlarged thyroid gland) or thyroid nodules • Heat intolerance • Increased appetite • Increased sweating • Itching - overall • Lack of menstrual periods in women • Nausea and vomiting • Pounding, rapid, or irregular pulse • Protruding eyes (exophthalmos)	• Clinical evalution • TFTs, thyroid scan • Glucose test • Radioactive iodine uptake
Cushing syndrome	(see 2.1.3 Endocrine) →17	
Primary hyperaldosteronism (Conn's disease)	• Hypertension • Muscle weakness • Polydipsia • Polyuria • Hypokalemia	• Blood test- Plasma aldosterone/renin ratio • 24-hour urinary excretion of aldosterone test • Serum electrolytes for hypokalemia • Saline suppression test of aldosterone

2.3   Polyuria (UO > 3000 ml/24h)

Probable Diagnosis	Symptoms/Signs	Diagnostic Procedures
CKD	(see 2.1.1 Renal) →15	
Diabetes insipidus (Central DI, Nephrogenic DI)	• Polyuria, polydipsia • Unexplained weakness • Lethargy • Muscle pains • Irritability	• UA • Fluid deprivation test • Serum sodium, urine sodium
Primary hyperaldosteronism	(see 2.2 Hypertension) →19	
Psychogenic or primary polydipsia	• Excessive water-drinking in the absence of a physiologic stimulus to drink • Polyuria • Anxiety • History of psychiatric illnesses	• Water deprivation test • Serum sodium and osmolality • Urinary osmolality and sodium
Diabetes mellitus, hyperglycemia	• Frequent urination • High blood glucose • High levels of sugar in the urine • Increased thirst • Headaches • Fatigue (weak, tired feeling)	• Blood sugar levels, HbA1c • Urine for ketones
Diuretics	• Recent initiation of diuretic for volume overload (eg, due to heart failure or peripheral edema) • Patients who are likely to surreptitiously use diuretics for weight loss (eg, those with eating disorders or concerns about weight, athletes, adolescents)	• Clinical evolution of volume status • Serum electrolytes and osmolality • Urine osmolality, sodium, potassium and chloride • Urine diuretic screen, if indicated

2.4   Hematuria

Probable Diagnosis	Symptoms/Signs	Diagnostic Procedures
Glomerulonephritis	(see 2.1.1 Renal) →15	
Urinary tract infection (UTI)	• Pain or burning upon urination • Urine is cloudy or smells bad • A strong, persistent urge to urinate • Passing frequent, small amounts of urine • Urine that appears red, bright pink or cola-colored – a sign of blood in the urine • Pelvic pain, in women	• UA, CBC • Urine and blood cultures • Pelvic exam in females • Vaginal discharge tested for STD organisms (for example, Neisseria and Chlamydia) • Special culture media • Urinary tract radiology when indicated
Kidney stone	• Flank pain, severe and colicky in nature • Pain often accompanied by restlessness, nausea and vomiting • Hematuria, gross or microscopic • Stone passage: May be felt but best to strain urine to catch stone	• Serum electrolytes, calcium, phosphate, creatinine • UA to look for hematuria, infection, crystals • Stone analysis • Noncontrast CT is preferable imaging • Abdominal x-ray (KUB), IVP or USG can be helpful, if CT unavailable
Bladder cancer	• Abdominal pain • Hematuria • Painful urination • Urinary frequency • Urinary urgency • Urine leakage (incontinence) • Weight loss • Fatigue	• Abdominal and pelvic CT scan, MRI scan • Cystoscopy • Bladder biopsy • UA, urine cytology

Hematuria (cont.)

Probable Diagnosis	Symptoms/Signs	Diagnostic Procedures
Drugs side effects or overdose [Aspirin, warfarin (Coumadin), or clopidogrel (Plavix)]	• Abdominal pain with cramping • Hematuria • Unusual bleeding (nose, mouth, vagina, or rectum) • Burning, itching, numbness, prickling, "pins and needles", or tingling feelings • Difficulty with breathing or swallowing • Dizziness, faintness, headache • Increased menstrual flow or vaginal bleeding	• History- warfarin overdose more common than other causes • Coagulation tests • Anatomical studies for causes are indicated even with anticoagulation hematuria • Clinical evaluation

2.5 Metallic Taste

Probable Diagnosis	Symptoms/Signs	Diagnostic Procedures
CKD	(see 2.1.1 Renal) →15	
Vitamin B-12 deficiency	• Tingling, numbness in fingers and toes • Weakness, tiredness or lightheadedness • Memory loss, disorientation, Depression • Loss of appetite • Palpitations and breathing • Sore tongue	• Clinical evaluation • CBC with differential and RBC MCV • Serum B12
Pregnancy	• Fatigue/tiredness • Nausea/morning sickness • Backaches • Headache • Frequent urination • Itchy skin during pregnancy, especially on the abdomen, thighs, breasts and arms	• Blood test: Pregnancy-associated plasma protein screening (PAPP-A), human chorionic gonadotropin (hCG) • Alpha-fetoprotein screening (AFP) • USG (abdominal+pelvis)

Metallic Taste (cont.)		
Probable Diagnosis	Symptoms/Signs	Diagnostic Procedures
Oral health and sinus problems (plaque, gingivitis, periodontitis, tooth decay and abscesses)	• Bleeding gums • Gums that are tender when touched, but otherwise painless • Mouth sores • Swollen gums	• Clinical evaluation • Dental X-rays
Drugs side effects or overdose (Clarithromycin, metronidazole, cisplatin, carboplatin, metformin)	• Nausea • Headaches • Loss of appetite • Rash	• Medical history • Blood testing as indicated

2.6   Weakness, Fatigue & Lethargy

Probable Diagnosis	Symptoms/Signs	Diagnostic Procedures
CKD	(see 2.1.1 Renal) →15	
Hypothyroidism	(see 2.1.3 Endocrine) →17	
Anemia	• Fatigue, lethargy, weakness • Dyspnea on exertion, progressing to dyspnea at rest • Lightheadedness • Dizziness • Fainting • Chest pain, angina • Palpitations	• Lab tests: CBC, Iron level, transferrin level, ferritin, vit B12, LFTs, folate, BUN, creatinine • Bone marrow biopsy • Normal lung examination • Systolic heart murmur may be present
Autoimmune disease	• Fatigue, lethargy, weakness • Fever • Malaise • Skin or joint findings	• CBC, CRP, ESR • Antinuclear antibody tests • Autoantibody tests
Depression	• Fatigue, lethargy, weakness • Feels helpless, hopeless • Loss of appetite • Anger • Irritability • Loathing of life	• Labs tests to rule out other medical conditions causing depression: TFT's, calcium, serum electrolytes, LFT's, BUN, creatinine • CT scan or MRI of the brain • EEG, ECG
Adrenal insufficiency (Addison's disease)	(See 2.9 Hyperkalemia)→25	

2.7 Shortness of Breath

Probable Diagnosis	Symptoms/Signs	Diagnostic Procedures
CKD	(see 2.1.1 Renal) →15	
Pneumonia	• Fever, chills, cough, purulent sputum • Dyspnea, tachycardia	• Chest x-ray
Pneumothorax	• Sometimtes unilateral diminished breath sounds • Subcutaneous air • May follow injury or occur spontaneously (especially in tall, thin patients or patients with COPD)	• Chest x-ray
Pulmonary embolism	• Pleuritic pain • Dyspnea, tachycardia, sometimes fever • Hemoptysis, shock	• CT angiography • V/Q scan • Doppler or duplex study of extremities showing positive findings of deep vein thrombosis
COPD exacerbation	• Cough • Poor air movement • Pursed lip breathing • Accessory muscle use for breathing	• Clinical evaluation • Chest x-ray • Arterial blood gasses (ABGs) • Pulmonary function testing
Asthma, bronchospasm, reactive airway disease	• Wheezing, poor air exchange • Arising spontaneously or after stimulus (eg, cold, exercise, allergen) • Sometimes pulsus paradoxus	• Clinical evaluation • Sometimes pulmonary function testing or bedside peak flow measurement
Foreign body inhalation	• Sudden cough or stridor	• Chest x-ray (inspiratory and expiratory) • Sometimes bronchoscopy
Restrictive lung disease	• Progressive dyspnea	• Chest x-ray • Pulmonary function testing
Interstitial lung disease	• Fine crackles on auscultation	• High-resolution chest CT (HRCT)

Shortness of Breath (cont.)		
Probable Diagnosis	Symptoms/signs	Diagnostic Procedures
Pleural effusion	• Pleuritic chest pain • Lung field that is dull to percussion • Diminished breath sounds	• Chest x-ray, Chest CT • Thoracentesis
CHF	(see 2.1.2 Cardiovascular) →16	
Anemia	(see 2.6 Weakness, Fatigue & Lethargy) →23	

2.8 Changes in Urination

Burning on Urination, Urgency and Frequency

Probable Diagnosis	Symptoms/Signs	Diagnostic Procedures
UTI	(see 2.4 Hematuria) →21	
Bladder cancer	(see 2.4 Hematuria) →21	
Interstitial cystitis (IC)	• Urgency • Frequency • Suprapubic pain • Dyspareunia	• UA • Cystoscopy • Biopsy of the bladder

2.9 Hyperkalemia

Probable Diagnosis	Symptoms/Signs	Diagnostic Procedures
CKD	(see 2.1.1 Renal) →15	
Acidosis	• Rapid breathing • Confusion • Lethargy • Shortness of breath	• ABGs • Serum electrolytes • Urine pH • PFTs • Chest x-ray
Glomerulonephritis	(see 2.4 Hematuria) →21	
Adrenal insufficiency (Addison's disease)	• Fatigue, weakness • Weight loss • GI symptoms • Hypotension • Hyperpigmentation • Hyponatremia • Hyperkalemia • Hypoglycemia	• Serum cortisol (morning or stressed) • Plasma ACTH (morning level) • Cosyntropin stimulation test
Hypoaldosteronism	Metabolic acidosis, nonanion gap with hyperkalemia	• Urine electrolytes and osm for TTKG & anion gap • Plasma renin, aldosterone and cortisol levels

2.10   Rash or Itchy, Dry Skin

Probable Diagnosis	Symptoms/Signs	Diagnostic Procedures
CKD	(see 2.1.1 Renal) →15	
Liver disease	• Nausea • Vomiting • Abdominal pain • Jaundice (a yellow discoloration of the skin) • Fatigue, weakness and weight loss • Itching due to deposits of bile salts	• LFTs, CBC, serum electrolytes, INR • Hepatitis viral serologic testing • Radiology - CT scan, USG, or MRI • Liver biopsy
Psoriasis	• Irritated, red, flaky patches of skin (dry and covered with silver, flaky scales) • Red patches may appear anywhere on the body, including the scalp • Pitting of fingernails • Joint pain	• Physical examination • Medical and family history • Skin biopsy • X-rays (if joint pains)
Eczema	• Blisters with oozing and crusting • Itchy and dry skin	• Medical and family history • Skin biopsy • Allergy skin testing
Pregnancy	(see 2.5 Metallic Taste) →22	
Drug allergy (antibiotics, antifungal, others)	• Red, itchy, and raised swellings on the skin • Fever • Muscle and joint aches	• Medical history • Blood testing, eg, eosinophil count • Skin biopsy

3   Renal Physiology

The kidney has multiple functions, including the following:

- Excretory function - elimination of small molecular "wastes" from the body
- Maintaining electrolyte balance
- Maintaining acid-base balance
- Maintaining appropriate body volumes and tonicity (osmolarity)
- Endocrine function - production of erythropoietin, renin, calcitriol and prostaglandins (not discussed here)
- Gluconeogenesis (not discussed here)

3.1   Anatomy of Kidney

Left Kidney

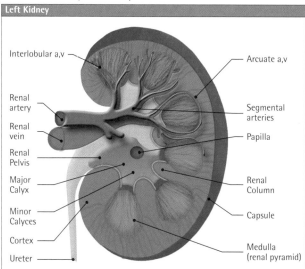

Interlobular a,v

Arcuate a,v

Renal artery

Segmental arteries

Renal vein

Papilla

Renal Pelvis

Major Calyx

Renal Column

Minor Calyces

Capsule

Cortex

Medulla (renal pyramid)

Ureter

3.2   Anatomy of a Nephron

Each kidney has about one million nephrons with a structure depicted in simplified fashion below. The nephrons are in close contact with the renal vasculature as the efferent arteriolar outflow of blood from the glomeruli perfuses the tubules in the kidney cortex. These arterioles form the vasa recta, capillary loops which extend into the renal medulla adjacent to the Loop of Henle and are important to maintain sodium reabsorption in the thick ascending limb necessary to both dilute the urine and maintain osmotic concentrations in the renal papillae needed to concentrate the urine.

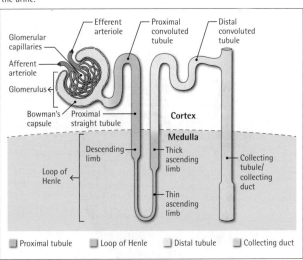

3.3   Physiology of Glomerular Filtration

- The renal blood flow is approximately 20% of the cardiac output at rest (1-1.2 L/min).
- The glomerular filtration rate (GFR) normally is approximately 120 ml/min or about 170-180 L/day.
- The filtration fraction, GFR/RPF (renal plasma flow), is approximately 20%, or about 10% of renal blood flow is filtered.
- GFR is determined by the pressure gradient across the glomerular capillary wall and basement membrane (GBM), the permeability of the GBM (filtration coefficient), and the filtration area.
- The pressure gradient driving glomerular filtration is the sum of the net hydraulic pressure (glomerular capillary hydrostatic pressure of ~55-60 mmHg less capsular hydrostatic pressure of ~15 mmHg or a net of ~40-45 mmHg) favoring filtration counteracted by the blood colloid osmotic pressure (~30 mmHg). As blood traverses the glomerular capillaries, filtration pressure equilibrium is reached as the fluid loss from the capillary lowers the hydraulic pressure and increases the colloid osmotic pressure as shown below.

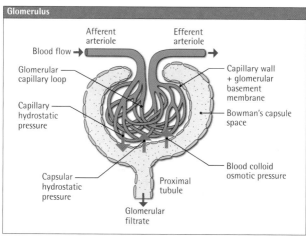

Glomerulus

The rate of glomerular filtration can be regulated by changing intraglomerular pressure, which is primarily regulated by changing the tonus of the afferent and efferent arterioles (ie, in the afferent arteriole, constriction reduces the flow and intraglomerular pressure, dilation increases the flow and intraglomerular pressure; whereas constriction of the efferent arteriole will increase intraglomerular pressure to maintain GFR even when blood flow is reduced).

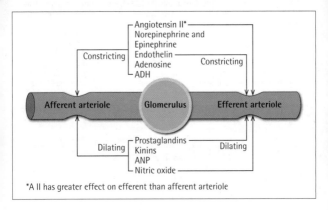

*A II has greater effect on efferent than afferent arteriole

3.4   Autoregulation of GFR

Autoregulation of GFR is a mechanism that maintains relatively constant renal blood flow and GFR despite changes in systemic arterial pressure. This mechanism fails at very low (MAP <50 mmHg) and very high (MAP >150 mmHg) arterial pressure, in which case renal blood flow, and to a lesser extent, GFR, decreases or increases, respectively. These autoregulatory factors, some of which are noted above, tend to maintain GFR at normal or near normal levels over a wide range of arterial blood pressures.

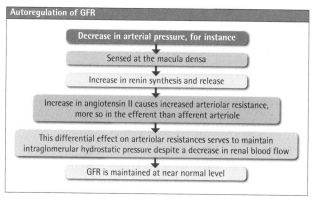

3.5   Tubular Function of the Nephron at a Glance

The glomerular filtrate of approximately 170-180 L/day allows the excretion of large quantities of small molecular waste products that are freely filtered and not reabsorbed by the tubules. The glomerular filtrate enters the renal tubules, and since the final urinary volume is about 1-1.5 L/day, about 99% of the fluid volume and the requisite amounts of electrolytes, glucose, amino acids, and proteins must be reabsorbed by the tubules to maintain body balance. This process depends upon the active renal tubular cell transport of sodium, an energy-requiring process that creates the osmotic and electrostatic forces which drive the reabsorptive transport of electrolytes and water and the secretion of other molecules, such as hydrogen ion, potassium, and uric acid. A general depiction of this function is shown below.

Renal Tubular Salt and Water Balance

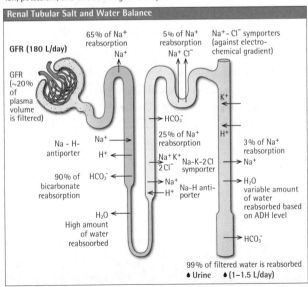

3.6 Renal Handling of Sodium

Under common conditions, over 99% of the filtered sodium is reabsorbed, primarily with bicarbonate and chloride as "accompanying" anions, or in the collecting ducts in exchange for secretion of hydrogen and potassium cations. The reabsorption of sodium and water to maintain homeostasis of body volumes is largely under the control of the GFR, glomerulotubular balance to increase or decrease sodium reabsorption in parallel with the GFR, and a number of regulatory hormones, the major ones of which are shown below.

Sodium Reabsorption in the Proximal Tubule

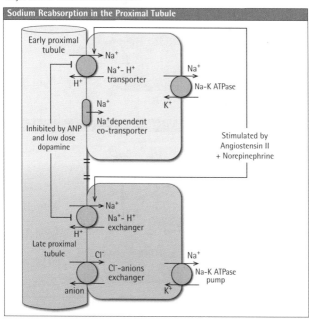

Sodium Reabsorption in the Loop of Henle

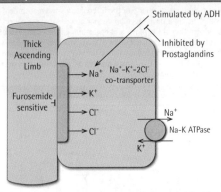

Sodium Reabsorption in the Distal Tubule

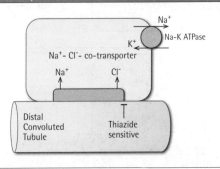

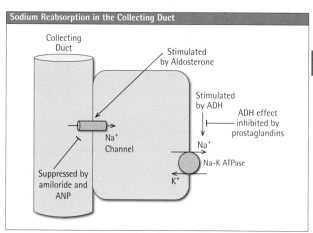

Sodium Reabsorption in the Collecting Duct

Collecting Duct

Stimulated by Aldosterone

Stimulated by ADH

ADH effect inhibited by prostaglandins

Na⁺ Channel

Na⁺

Na-K ATPase

K⁺

Suppressed by amiloride and ANP

Kidney Regulation of Sodium Balance

Mechanism of increased sodium reabsorption

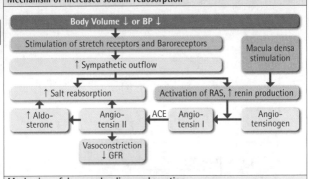

Body Volume ↓ or BP ↓

Stimulation of stretch receptors and Baroreceptors

↑ Sympathetic outflow

Macula densa stimulation

↑ Salt reabsorption

Activation of RAS, ↑ renin production

↑ Aldo-sterone ← Angio-tensin II ← ACE ← Angio-tensin I ← Angio-tensinogen

Vasoconstriction ↓ GFR

Mechanism of decreased sodium reabsorption

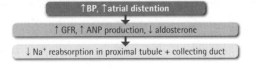

↑ BP, ↑ atrial distention

↑ GFR, ↑ ANP production, ↓ aldosterone

↓ Na^+ reabsorption in proximal tubule + collecting duct

3.7 Acid–base Regulation

To maintain normal blood pH, the kidney must first reabsorb the filtered bicarbonate. This takes place mainly in the proximal tubule in a process largely coupled to sodium reabsorption and hydrogen ion (H^+) secretion which is dependent upon carbonic anhydrase by the mechanisms shown below. Since most human diets produce metabolic acids to excrete, after reabsorption of bicarbonate takes place, additional hydrogen ions are secreted into the urine to be excreted as "titratable" acid at urine pH levels that can be reduced below 5 and by ammonium ions. Alkalinization of the urine by bicarbonate secretion, though also shown below, can take place but is usually unnecessary.

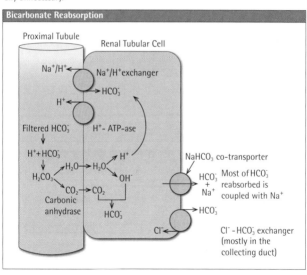

Bicarbonate Secretion

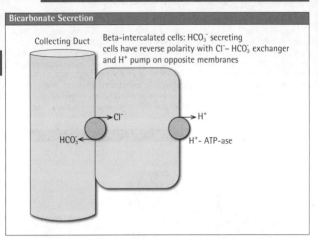

Collecting Duct

Beta-intercalated cells: HCO_3^- secreting cells have reverse polarity with Cl^-–HCO_3^- exchanger and H^+ pump on opposite membranes

Cl^-

HCO_3^-

H^+

H^+- ATP-ase

3.8   Renal Acid Excretion

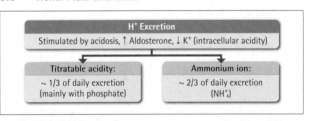

H⁺ Excretion
Stimulated by acidosis, ↑ Aldosterone, ↓ K⁺ (intracellular acidity)

Titratable acidity:	Ammonium ion:
~ 1/3 of daily excretion (mainly with phosphate)	~ 2/3 of daily excretion (NH_4^+)

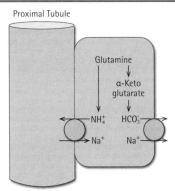

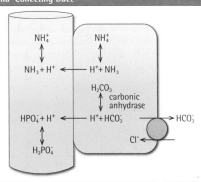

3.9   Potassium Homeostasis

Total body stores of potassium amount to about 3000 mEq, most of which is intracellular, as in muscle cells, and in bone while only about 60 mEq or 2% of potassium is in the extracellular fluid. Since maintenance of the potassium electrical gradient across heart muscle cell membranes is so important, precise regulation of potassium distribution between the intracellular and extracellular fluid compartments is essential. The major factors increasing cellular uptake of potassium are insulin and betasympathetic catecholamines (epinephrine) which stimulate Na-K ATPase and alkalosis with low intracellular H^+ ion that will lower serum K^+, or the opposite wherein low insulin, alpha sympathetic catecholamines, or acidosis will raise serum K^+ as shown below.

In addition, the ultimate regulation of total body potassium depends upon renal excretion of the approximately 100 mEq/day of potassium ingested in the diet to maintain proper potassium balance. About 90% of the roughly 700 mEq/day of potassium filtered by the glomeruli is reabsorbed and then in the distal nephron, most of the remainder may be absorbed to conserve potassium, or more commonly, potassium is secreted into the collecting duct to excrete excess potassium. The major factors affecting potassium excretion are aldosterone, distal tubular Na^+ delivery, urine flow rate, and acid-base status as shown below. In addition, potassium adaptation stimulated by increased K^+ in the diet or high serum K^+ causes both increased intracellular uptake of K^+ by muscle cells and increased renal K^+ excretion to protect against worsening hyperkalemia (with the opposite in cases of low K^+ diets and low serum K^+ levels to protect against hypokalemia).

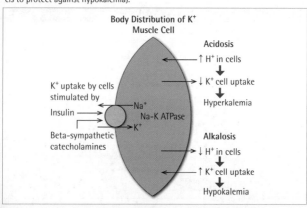

Renal Handling of K⁺

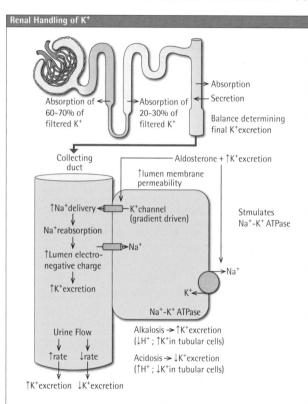

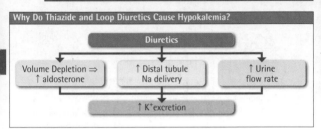

Why Do Thiazide and Loop Diuretics Cause Hypokalemia?

3.10   Diuretic Sites of Action in the Nephron

The three major classes of diuretics used for enhancing sodium excretion are **thiazide diuretics, loop diuretics, and potassium-sparing diuretics** (either aldosterone antagonists or sodium channel blockers). Other drugs have diuretic action, but are used for more specific purposes, such as carbonic anhydrase inhibitors (to cause bicarbonaturia or alkalinize the urine), osmotic diuretics (to enhance urinary excretion of poisons or for CNS edema), low-dose dopamine (for CHF and AKI, but probably no longer indicated for AKI treatment) and ADH antagonists (to induce a water diuresis to correct hyponatremia). Their sites of action in the renal tubule are shown in the diagram below.

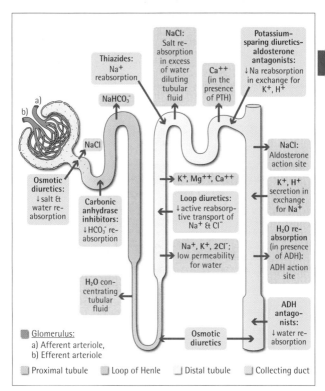

3.11   Renal Handling of Calcium

Since calcium is partially bound to albumin, about 6 mg/dL of calcium is filtered, amounting to about 10,800 mg/day in the 180 L/day of glomerular filtrate. With intestinal absorption, and therefore, renal excretion amounting to about 200 mg/day, 98% of the filtered calcium is reabsorbed by the tubules. In the proximal tubule and the Loop of Henle, about 80% of the calcium is reabsorbed, largely paralleling sodium reabsorption. In the distal tubule where about 15% of the calcium is reabsorbed, hormonal regulation controls calcium reabsorption to achieve body balance by the mechanisms shown below.

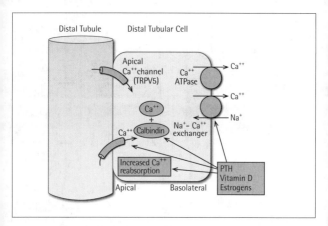

3.12 Renal Handling of Phosphate

Phosphate is filtered at the glomerulus and reabsorbed mainly in the proximal tubule with a fractional excretion of about 15-20% commonly, but which is quite variable depending upon dietary phosphate intake. Tubular reabsorption is under the regulation of the hormones PTH and FGF 23, which exert a phosphaturic action by blocking phosphate reabsorption as shown below.

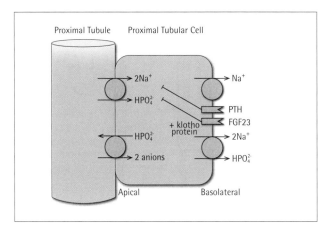

3.13   Renal Handling of Water

A simplified schema of the tubular water reabsorption mechanisms to reduce the urine volume to approximately 1% of the filtered fluid volume are depicted here. One mechanism is the passive water reabsorption in the proximal tubule, Loop of Henle, and distal tubule based on the isosmolar cortical and hyperosmolar medullary environments and the second is the ADH-dependent water reabsorption mainly in the collecting duct to determine the final urine concentration.

Passive Water Reabsorption

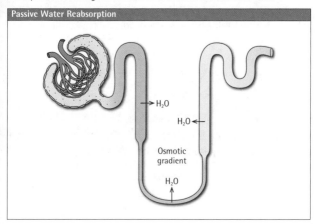

ADH – Mediated Water Reabsorption

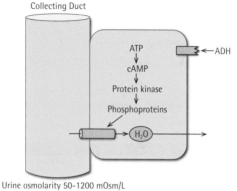

Collecting Duct

ATP
↓
cAMP
↓
Protein kinase
↓
Phosphoproteins

H_2O

← ADH

Urine osmolarity 50-1200 mOsm/L
ADH ↓ ☐➔ ↑

ADH increases water reabsorption and urine osmolarity

References and Suggested Reading

Danziger J, Zeidel M, Parker MJ. Renal physiology: A clinical approach. Lippincott Williams & Wilkins, Philadelphia, 2012

Rose BD, Post TW. Clinical physiology of acid-base and electrolyte disorders, 5th ed, McGraw-Hill, New York, 2001

Schrier RW. Renal and electrolyte disorders, 7th ed, Lippincott Williams & Wilkins, Philadelphia, 2010

Rennke HG, Denker, BM. Renal pathophysiology: The essentials, 3rd ed, Lippincott Williams & Wilkins, Philadelphia, 2009

Eaton D, Pooler J. Vanders renal physiology, 8th ed, McGraw-Hill, New York, 2013

Jameson J, Loscalzo J. Harrison's nephrology and acid-base disorders, McGraw-Hill, New York, 2010

Deen WM, Bridges CR, Brenner BM, Myers BD. Heteroporous model of glomerular size selectivity: application to normal and nephrotic humans. Am J Physiol 1985; 249: F374-89.

Lambers TT, Bindels RJ, Hoenderop JG. Coordinated control of renal Ca^{2+} handling. Kidney Internat 2006; 69(2): 650-4

Eladari D, Chambrey R, Peti-Peterdi J. A new look at electrolyte transport in the distal tubule. Annu Rev Physiol 2012; 74:325-49..

4   Urinalysis and Diagnostic Tests

4.1   Urinalysis

The clinician has an invaluable tool in the evaluation of patients by the examination of the urine. Easy to obtain, but often overlooked, the voided urine offers clues to the diagnosis of kidney conditions and help with the prognosis in cardiovascular disease and diabetes.

A complete urinalysis consists of visual inspection for color and turbidity, a dipstick exam, and a microscopic exam of the centrifuged urinary sediment. While the dipstick is a "waived" test that can be done in any office, the microscopic exam requires Clinical Laboratory Improvement Amendments (CLIA) certification so it would usually be performed by a clinical laboratory, nephrologist, or a trained physician or technician.

4.2   Urine Color

Color	Causes	
Cloudy or turbid	• Pyuria • Bacteriuria	• Heavy crystalluria • Fecal or vaginal contamination
White	• WBCs	• Chyle
Red or cola-colored	• RBCs (supernatant may be clear) • Free hemoglobin (Hgb) • Myoglobin • Porphyria (porphobilin & porphyrins) **Dye** • Phenolphthalein	**Food** • Cascara • Senna • Beets **Drugs** • Doxorubicin • Phenazopyridine • Phenytoin
Yellow	**Vitamin supplement** • Riboflavin	**Dye** • Yellow Dye
Dark yellow/orange	**Drugs** • Sulfasalazine • Rifampin	• Bilirubin
Black/brown	**Drugs** • Methyldopa • Levodopa • Metronidazole • Imipenem-cilastatin	**Other** • Melanin **Condition** • Homogentisic acid (alkaptonuria)

Urine Color (cont.)	Causes	
Dull blue/green	**Drugs** • Triamterene • Amitriptyline • Propofol	**Drug/dye** • Methylene blue **Infection** • Pseudomonas UTI
	Endogenous metabolite: Biliverdin	

4.3   Dipstick Test

Dipstick	Positive	False Positive	False Negative
Blood	Detects RBCs as low as 1-2/hpf, but also reacts to free hemoglobin (hemolysis) and myoglobin (rhabdomyolysis)	Uncommon - contamination with hypochlorite or bacteria with pseudoperoxidase activity	Rare - high concentration of ascorbic acid can mask low-grade hematuria
Proteins	Detects albumin >30 mg/dL (normal is negative; trace - 27% will have microalbuminuria; 1+ - 47 % will have micro- or macro-albuminuria)	Highly buffered alkaline urine, some antiseptics, such as chlorhexidine, ejaculation	Light chains & other immunoglobulins, beta-2-microglobulin, dilute urine with <30 mg/dl of albumin
Nitrites	Denotes Enterobacteriaceae which convert urinary nitrate to nitrite in UTI	None	Short incubation time in the bladder (<4 hours), pathogen doesn't convert nitrate to nitrite, not enough nitrate or too much ascorbic acid in urine
Leukocyte esterase	Detects pyuria ≥6 WBCs/hpf but may indicate interstitial nephritis or leukemia rather than infection	Contamination with vaginal discharge or saliva	High glucose or specific gravity, some antibiotics, only mononuclear leukocytes in transplant rejection

Dipstick	Positive	False Positive	False Negative
Glucose	Detects diabetes and renal glucosuria	None	Ascorbic acid or ketones in urine decreases positive tests
Ketones	Detects acetoacetate in diabetic and starvation/alcoholic ketosis	High quantities of levodopa or mesna in urine	Doesn't detect acetone or beta-hydroxybutyrate ketone bodies

4.4 Proteinuria

4.4.1 Protein to creatinine ratio (PCR) and albumin to creatinine ratio (ACR)

Estimation of the degree of proteinuria in a random or spot urine

Urine protein to creatinine ratio measures all proteins and is calculated as:

$$\frac{U_{protein} \ (mg/dL)}{U_{creatinine} \ (mg/dL)} = \frac{protein \ (gm)}{creatinine \ (gm)}$$

This correlates with grams of protein excreted per day per 1.73 m^2 body surface area (BSA).

Detect micro- or macro–albuminuria in a random or spot urine

Urine albumin to creatinine ratio is calculated as:

$$\frac{U_{albumin} \ (mg/L)}{U_{creatinine} \ (gm/L)} = \frac{albumin \ (mg)}{creatinine \ (gm)}$$

Proteinuria	Prot/Cr ratio on spot urine	24-hour urine collection
Normal	<0.2 (usually unit-free but can be gm/gm)	<150 mg/24h
Mild proteinuria	0.2 – 1.0	150 mg – 1.0 gm/24h
Moderate proteinuria	1.0 – 3.0	1.0 – 3.0 gm/24h
Nephrotic range	>3.0	>3.0 gm/24h

Albuminuria	Alb/Cr ratio on spot urine	24-hour urine collection
Normal	<30 mg/gm is considered normal but gender-based normals are: <17 mg/gm (men) <25 mg/gm (women)	<30 mg/24h
Microalbuminuria	30 - 300 mg/gm (either sex) or 17 - 300 mg/gm (men) 25 - 300 mg/gm (women)	30 - 300 mg/24h
Macroalbuminuria	>300 mg/gm	>300 mg/24h

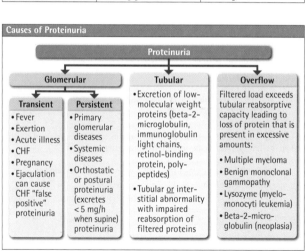

Causes of Proteinuria

Proteinuria

Glomerular

Transient
• Fever
• Exertion
• Acute illness
• CHF
• Pregnancy
• Ejaculation can cause CHF "false positive" proteinuria

Persistent
• Primary glomerular diseases
• Systemic diseases
• Orthostatic or postural proteinuria (excretes <5 mg/h when supine) proteinuria

Tubular
• Excretion of low-molecular weight proteins (beta-2-microglobulin, immunoglobulin light chains, retinol-binding protein, poly-peptides)
• Tubular or inter-stitial abnormality with impaired reabsorption of filtered proteins

Overflow
Filtered load exceeds tubular reabsorptive capacity leading to loss of protein that is present in excessive amounts:
• Multiple myeloma
• Benign monoclonal gammopathy
• Lysozyme (myelo-monocyti leukemia)
• Beta-2-micro-globulin (neoplasia)

4.5   Estimation of Renal Function

Measured creatinine clearance (C_{Cr}):

Collect timed urine for volume and total creatinine excretion (usually 24h collection in which total urine volume is divided by 1440 min/24 h in the formula below)

> Normal daily Cr excretion: – Males: 15–20 mg/Kg/24h
> – Females: 10–15 mg/Kg/24h
> Creatinine clearance ml/min = $\dfrac{U_{Cr}\ (mg/dL)\ x\ U_{Vol}\ (ml/min)}{S_{Cr}\ (mg/dL)}$

Measured glomerular filtration rate (GFR):
Rarely done except for research studies:
• Inulin clearance
• I^{125}- iothalamate clearance

Estimated creatinine clearance calculated from serum creatinine:

Cockcroft Gault formula

> $$eC_{Cr}\ (ml/min) = \frac{(140 - age)}{S_{Cr}\ (mg/dL)}\ x\ \frac{Body\ weight\ (Kg)}{72}\ x\ (0.85\ if\ female)$$

Original formula used actual body weight (BW), but to avoid overestimate of eC_{Cr} if weight is >120% of ideal body weight (IBW), it is better to use:

> **Either IBW or 0.4 (BW – IBW) + IBW where IBW is calculated as:**
> • IBW for women (Kg) = 45 + (2.3 x inches over 60")
> • IBW for men (Kg)   = 50 + (2.3 x inches over 60")

Cockcroft DW, Gault MH. Prediction of creatinine clearance from serum creatinine. *Nephron.* 1976;16(1):31-41.

Estimated glomerular filtration rate calculated from serum creatinine:

The CKD-EPI (Chronic Kidney Disease Epidemiology Collaboration) equation for eGFR has updated the various MDRD formulae, as more accurate particularly with GFRs in the range over 60 mL/min per 1.73 m^2. However, many experts favor reporting only that eGFR >60 mL/min per 1.73 m^2 for "normal" eGFRs due to lack of accuracy in this range.

$$eGFR =$$
$$141 \times \min (Scr/\kappa,1)^{\alpha} \times \max (Scr/\kappa,1)^{-1.209} \times 0.993^{Age} \times 1.018 \text{ [if female]} \times 1.159 \text{ [if black]}$$

Where Scr is standardized serum creatinine (mg/dL), κ is 0.7 for females and 0.9 for males, α is −0.329 for females and −0.411 for males, min indicates the minimum of Scr/κ or 1, and max indicates the maximum of Scr/κ or 1

Levey AS, Stevens LA, Schmid CH, et al. A new equation to estimate glomerular filtration rate. *Ann Intern Med* 2009;150(9):604–612.

Calculator for eGFR in adults, children or PDA is at:
http://www.kidney.org/professionals/kdoqi/gfr.cfm

Osmolality to Specific Gravity

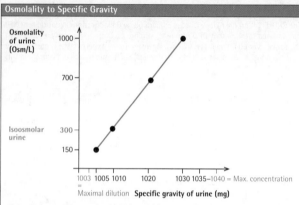

Note: Presence of dense molecules in the urine (glucose, radiocontrast media, heavy proteinuria) can produce large changes in specific gravity (SG) with relatively little change in osmolality so SG should not be used to estimate osmolality in such cases.

4.6   Urine Sediment Findings

| Urine Sediment Findings | | |
Cells	Casts	Crystals (see →172)

• **Red blood cells**: Hematuria may be of non-glomerular or glomerular origin, the latter indicated by acanthocytic RBCs or RBC casts
• **White blood cells**:
  – Polymorphs (pyuria in UTI)
  – Eosinophils (need staining to identify)
  – Lymphocytes (in acute transplant rejection or interstitial nephritis)
  – Macrophages (uncertain significance)
• **Epithelial cells**:
  – Renal tubular cells (ATN, nephrotic syndrome, transplant rejection, interstitial nephritis)
  – Squamous epithelial cells (may signify vaginal contamination)
  – Transitional cells (bladder, ureters, or renal pelvis origin - usually benign but can be malignant)
• **Bacteria, fungi or parasites**
	Organic matrix composed primarily of Tamm-Horsfall mucoprotein (also called uromodulin)
	• **Hyaline casts**: Not indicative of disease, observed with small volumes of concentrated urine or with diuretic therapy
	• **Red blood cell casts**: Diagnostic of glomerulonephritis or vasculitis
	• **White blood cell casts**: Pyelonephritis, acute glomerulonephritis, tubulointerstitial disease
	• **Epithelial cell casts**: Acute tubular necrosis and rarely in acute glomerulonephritis
	• **Lipid or fatty casts**: Nephrotic-range proteinuria (the degeneration of lipid-laden renal tubular cells in the casts may result in characteristic "Maltese cross" droplets composed of cholesterol esters and cholesterol, which may also be observed as free fat or as oval fat bodies in the urine).
	• **Granular casts**: Observed in numerous disorders, represent degenerating cells or aggregated proteins in casts
	• **Waxy casts**: Represent the last stage of the degeneration of granular casts.
	• **Broad casts**: May be waxy or granular and form in the enlarged tubules of nephrons that have hypertrophied in advanced renal failure.
		• **Uric acid crystals**: Observed in acid urine from the conversion of the more soluble urate salt into less soluble uric acid
		• **Calcium phosphate**: Form in a relatively alkaline urine
		• **Calcium oxalate**: Most common crystal and kidney stone, not dependent upon the urine pH
		• **Cystine crystals**: Seen only in cystinuria
		• **Triple phosphate crystals**: Magnesium ammonium phosphate crystals + calcium carbonate-apatite = struvite or "triple phosphate" crystals (occurs only when ammonia production is increased and the urine pH is elevated to decrease the solubility of phosphate in the setting of urease-producing organisms such as Proteus or Klebsiella).
		• **Drug crystals**: Mainly acyclovir, indinavir, atazanavir, triamterene, methotrexate, sulfonamide antibiotics

4.7   Hematuria

Hematuria is defined (arbitrarily) as presence of ≥2-3 RBC per high powered field (hpf) in spun urine.

4.7.1   Classification & Causes

The amount determines whether it is visible to naked eye or requires microscopy for detection:

- Macroscopic (or gross) hematuria
- Microscopic hematuria

Causes of Hematuria	
Urologic diseases (non-glomerular and usually without proteinuria)	

• **Transient hematuria:**
  - Most common cause of hematuria is infection (cystitis, prostatitis, or pyelonephritis)
  - Trauma, exercise
  - Menstruation
  - Sexual intercourse
	• **Persistent hematuria:**
	  - Neoplasms
	  - Nephrolithiasis
	  - Hypercalciuria or hyperuricosuria
	  - Renal cystic disease
	  - Tuberculosis

Hematologic disorders	
• Sickle cell trait or disease • Coagulopathies, particularly high INR • Hemolytic uremic syndrome/thrombotic thrombocytopenic purpura (HUS/TTP)	
Glomerular disorders	

• Signs of glomerular origin: red blood cell casts, acanthocytes, and dysmorphic RBCs, proteinuria >500 mg/d, cola-colored urine
• Persistent hematuria:
  - Any glomerular disease, but more common in acute nephritic disease
  - IgA nephropathy
  - Hereditary nephritis (Alport's syndrome)
  - Thin basement membrane disease
  - Renal vasculitis	

Other	
• Vascular disease • Systemic vasculitis • Renal infarction • AV malformation, renal angiomas	• AV fistula • Malignant hypertension • Papillary necrosis • Loin pain hematuria syndrome

4.7.2   Hematuria Evaluation

- Examine urinary sediment for glomerular etiology
- Radiologic imaging for renal anatomy (tumor mass, stones, polycystic kidneys, hydronephrosis, AV malformation, medullary sponge kidney, kidney size)
  - Ultrasound — safe, can be used in pregnancy, less expensive
  - Intravenous pyelography (IVP) — readily available, shows ureters, poor differentiation of solid vs cystic masses, less expensive than CT, but should probably be used only if other studies are not available
  - CT scan (without than with radiocontrast) — best for stones and masses, can show vasculature and detect some bladder tumors
  - MRI (without and with gadolinium) — equal to CT for masses and vasculature, less risk of contrast toxicity but can't use in stage 4 or 5 CKD due to risk of gadolinium nephrogenic systemic fibrosis
  - Renal arteriography — if CT suggests infarction or AV malformation
  - Retrograde or percutaneous antegrade pyelography — to evaluate obstruction in hydronephrosis
- Cystoscopy (bladder mass or stone, unresolving cystitis) — indicated in gross hematuria or persistent non-glomerular microscopic hematuria in patients over 40 – 50 years old or with risk factors for transitional cell cancer
- Urine cytology — can detect transitional cell cancer with high specificity but low sensitivity, not useful for renal cell cancer
- Renal biopsy — low yield unless proteinuria, renal insufficiency, or clinical evidence of glomerular disease

4.8   Eosinophiluria

Detect with Hansel's stain of the urinary sediment
- Allergic interstitial nephritis
- Acute prostatitis or UTI
- Atheroembolic disease
- Occasionally vasculitis or rapidly progressive glomerulonephritis
- Transplant rejection

4.9 Kidney Biopsy

4.9.1 Indications for kidney biopsy

- **Acute renal failure:** Rising creatinine when cause is unclear or >3–4 weeks of supportive Rx without recovery
- **Acute nephritic syndrome**, progressive renal insufficiency
- **Proteinuria:** Without evidence of known causative systemic disease: Nephrotic syndrome or >1–2 g/day non-nephrotic range proteinuria to determine diagnosis and prognosis
- **Hematuria:** Recurrent gross hematuria or persistent microscopic hematuria of suspected renal etiology or family Hx of hematuria when Dx would help management
- **Systemic disease:** Systemic lupus erythematosus (SLE) or systemic vasculitis with renal findings, undiagnosed systemic disease, or atypical course of diabetic nephropathy
- **Transplant kidney:** Allograft dysfunction to differentiate ATN vs transplant rejection vs drug toxicity vs viral interstitial nephritis vs recurrent or de novo glomerulonephritis vs thrombotic microangiopathy

4.9.2 Relative contraindications for biopsy

- Anatomic abnormalities: eg, solitary, ectopic, cystic, or horseshoe kidney may be more effectively biopsied using CT rather than US localization
- Uncorrected coagulation disorders and thrombocytopenia.
- Uremic platelet dysfunction is a relative contraindication that may be helped by DDAVP pre-treatment
- Severe uncontrolled HTN
- Active renal or perirenal bacterial infection should preclude biopsy until controlled with Rx
- Hydronephrosis
- Small kidneys (<9 cm) in an adult is usually indicative of chronic irreversible disease
- Impaired mental status or uncooperative patient will necessitate sedation for safety

4.9.3 Complications of biopsy

- Gross hematuria occurs in 3% –10% and is usually self-limited
- Hematuria or perinephric bleeding that causes hypotension occurs in 1% – 2%
- Bleeding requiring blood transfusion occurs in 1% – 2%
- Infection is rare unless UTI is present pre-biopsy
- AV fistula formation is rare but may cause persistent hematuria and a renal bruit
- Death occurs in about 1 in 8000 biopsies (more frequently in other studies – 0.1%)
- An observation period of ≤8 h risks missing ≥20% – 33% of complications

References and Suggested Reading

Urinalysis and Diagnostic Tests

Fogazzi GB, Verdesca S, Garigali G. Urinalysis: core curriculum. Am J Kidney Dis. 2008 Jun 51(6):1052-67

Cockcroft D.W., Gault M.H. Prediction of creatinine clearance from serum creatinine. Nephron. 1976;16:31-41

Levey, A.S., et al. A More Accurate Method To Estimate Glomerular Filtration rate from Serum Creatinine: A New Prediction Equation. Ann Intern Med. 1999; 130 (6):461-470

Levey AS, Coresh J, Greene T, et al. Using standardized serum creatinine values in the modification of diet in renal disease study equation for estimating glomerular filtration rate. Ann Intern Med. 2006;145(4):247-254.

Schwartz GJ, Muñoz A, Schneider MF, et al. New equations to estimate GFR in children with CKD. J Am Soc Nephrol. 2009; 20(3):629–37.

Levey AS, Stevens LA, Schmid CH, et al. A new equation to estimate glomerular filtration rate. Ann Intern Med 2009;150(9):604-612.

Matsushita K, Mahmoodi BK, Woodward M, et al. Comparison of risk prediction using the CKD-EPI equation and the MDRD study equation for estimated glomerular filtration rate. JAMA 2012; 307(18):1941-51.

Hematuria

Vivante, et al. Persistent asymptomatic isolated microscopic hematuria in Israeli adolescents and young adults and risk for end-stage renal disease. JAMA 306:729-736; 2011

Cohen RA, Brown RS. Microscopic hematuria. New Engl J Med 348: 2330-2338, 2003.

Grossfeld GD, et al. Asymptomatic Microscopic Hematuria in Adults: Summary of the AUA Best Practice Policy Recommendations. Am Fam Physician. 2001;63:1145-1155.

Andres A, et. al.; Hematuria due to hypercalciuria and hyperuricosuria in adult patients. Kidney Int 36:96-99, 1989.

Chow, KM, Kwan, BC, Li, PK, Szeto, CC. Asymptomatic isolated microscopic haematuria: long-term follow-up. QJM 2004; 97:739.

Khadra MH, Pickard RS, Charlton M, Powell PH, Neal DE. A prospective analysis of 1,930 patients with hematuria to evaluate current diagnostic practice. J Urol 2000;163:524-7

Offringa M, Benbassat J. The value of urinary red cell shape in the diagnosis of glomerular and post-glomerular haematuria-a meta-analysis. Postgrad Med J 1992;68:648-54.

Kitamoto Y, et al. Differentiation of hematuria using a uniquely shaped red cell. Nephron 1993; 64:32-36.

Kohler H, et al. Acanthocyturia-a characteristic marker for glomerular bleeding. Kidney Int 1991;40:115-20

Hall, CL, Bradley, R, Kerr, A, et al. Clinical value of renal biopsy in patients with asymptomatic microscopic hematuria with and without low-grade proteinuria. Clin Nephrol 2004; 62:267.

Britton, JP, et al.: Dipstick haematuria and bladder cancer in men over 60: Results of a community study. BMJ 299:1010, 1989.

Copley JB: Idiopathic hematuria: A prospective evaluation. Arch Intern Med 147:434-437,1987.

Culclasure, TF, et al.; The significance of hematuria in the anticoagulated patient. Arch Intern Med:154:649, 1994

Hiatt RA, Ordonez JD. Dipstick urinalysis screening, asymptomatic microhematuria, and subsequent urological cancers in a population-based sample. Cancer Epidemiol Biomarkers Prev 1994;3:439-43

McGregor DO, et al. Clinical audit of the use of renal biopsy in the management of microscopic hematuria. Clincal Nephrology 1998;49:345-8.

References and Suggested Reading (cont.)

Hematuria (cont.)

Siegel AJ, et al: Exercise-related hematuria: Findings in a group of marathon runners. JAMA 241:391-392, 1979

Tiebosch ATMG, et al. Thin-basement-membrane nephropathy in adults with persistent hematuria. N Engl J Med 1989;320:14-8.

Topham PS, et al. Glomerular disease as a cause of isolated microscopic haematuria. Q J Med 1994; 87:329-35

Van Savage JG, Fried FA. Anticoagulant associated hematuria: a prospective study. J Urol 1995;153: 1594-6.

Feifer AH, et al. Utility of urine cytology in the workup of asymptomatic microscopic hematuria in low-risk patients. Urology 2010;75:1278-82.

Proteinuria

Brown RS. Has the time come to include urine dipstick testing in screening asymptomatic young adults? JAMA 306 ; 2011

Wen CP, Yang YC, Tsai MK. Urine dipstick to detect proteinuria: An unused tool for an underappreciated risk marker. Am J Kidney Dis 2011;58(1):1-3.

White SL, et al. Diagnostic accuracy of urine dipsticks for detection of albuminuria in the general community. Am J Kidney Dis 2011;58(1):19-28.

Clark WF, Macnab JJ, Sontrop JM, Jain AK, Moist L, Salvadori M, et al; Dipstick proteinuria as a screening strategy to identify rapid renal decline. J Am Soc Nephrol 2011;22(9):1729-36

Boulware, LE, Jaar, BG, Tarver-Carr, ME, et al. Screening for proteinuria in US adults: a cost-effectiveness analysis. JAMA 2003; 290:3101.

Keane WF. Proteinuria: its clinical importance and role in progressive renal disease. Am J Kidney Dis. 2000; 35 (4 Suppl 1):S97-105.

Schwab, SJ, Christensen, RL, Dougherty, K, Klahr, S. Quantitation of proteinuria by the use of protein-to-creatinine ratios in single urine samples. Arch Intern Med 1987; 147:943.

Bennett PH, et al.: Screening and management of microalbuminuria in patients with diabetes mellitus: Recommendations to the Scientific Advisory Board of the NKF. Am J Kidney Dis 25:107-112,1995.

Ginsberg JSM, et al.; Use of single voided urine samples to estimate quantitative proteinuria. N Engl J Med 309:1543-1546, 1983.

Springberg, PD, Garrett, LE Jr, Thompson, AL, et al. Fixed and reproducible orthostatic proteinuria: Results of a 20-year follow-up study. Ann Intern Med 1982; 97:516.

Cirillo M Lanti MP Menotti A et al. Definition of kidney dysfunction as a cardiovascular risk factor: use of urinary albumin excretion and estimated glomerular filtration rate. Arch Intern Med 2008; 168: 617-24.

Renal Biopsy

National Kidney Foundation information about kidney biopsy: http://www.kidney.org.uk/Medical-Info/kidney-disease/biopsy.html#7. Last accessed on March 21, 2012.

Atwell TD, Smith RL, Hesley GK, et al. Incidence of bleeding after 15,181 percutaneous biopsies and the role of aspirin. Am J Roentgenol (AJR) 2010;194:784-9.

Hergesell O, Felten H, Andrassy K, Kuhn K, Ritz E. Safety of ultrasound-guided percutaneous renal biopsy-retrospective analysis of 1090 consecutive cases. Nephrol Dial Transplant 1998;13:975-7.

Manno C, Strippoli GF, Arnesano L, et al. Predictors of bleeding complications in percutaneous ultrasound-guided renal biopsy. Kidney Int. 2004;66:1570-7.

References and Suggested Reading (cont.)

Renal Biopsy

Marwah DS, Korbet SM. Timing of complications in percutaneous renal biopsy: what is the optimal period of observation? Am J Kidney Dis 1996;28:47-52.

Whittier WL, Korbet SM. Timing of complications in percutaneous renal biopsy. J Am Soc Nephrol 2004;15:142-7.

Whittier WL, Korbet SM. Renal biopsy: update. Curr Opin Nephrol Hypertens 2004;13:661-5

5 Water and Electrolyte Disorders

5.1 Water Distribution Between Body Compartments

The diagram below illustrates water distribution between different body ompartments: Intracellular and extracellular, the latter including interstitial and intravascular spaces.

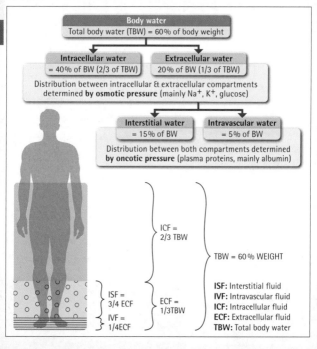

5.2 Sites of Electrolyte Reabsorption

The simplified diagram below illustrates important sites of electrolyte reabsorption in the nephron and where Na^+ reabsorption can be inhibited by diuretics.

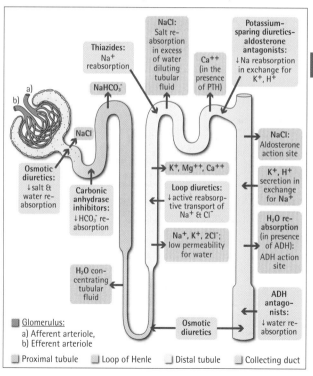

5.3   Hypernatremia

Causes of hypernatremia are divided into three categories based on the patient's volume status. Hypernatremia is not very frequent (0.1% - 0.2% of hospitalized patients). It is always associated with hypertonicity (hyperosmolality).

Hypernatremia: Causes

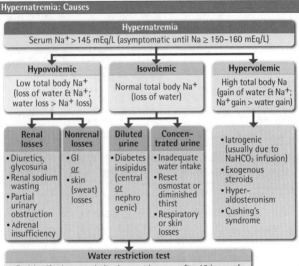

Hypernatremia
Serum Na^+ > 145 mEq/L (asymptomatic until Na ≥ 150–160 mEq/L)

Hypovolemic
Low total body Na^+
(loss of water & Na^+; water loss > Na^+ loss)

Isovolemic
Normal total body Na^+
(loss of water)

Hypervolemic
High total body Na
(gain of water & Na^+; Na^+ gain > water gain)

Renal losses
- Diuretics, glycosuria
- Renal sodium wasting
- Partial urinary obstruction
- Adrenal insufficiency

Nonrenal losses
- GI
  or
- skin (sweat) losses

Diluted urine
- Diabetes insipidus (central or nephrogenic)

Concentrated urine
- Inadequate water intake
- Reset osmostat or diminished thirst
- Respiratory or skin losses

- Iatrogenic (usually due to $NaHCO_3$ infusion)
- Exogenous steroids
- Hyper-aldosteronism
- Cushing's syndrome

Water restriction test
Positive if urine osmolarity does not increase after 12 hours of water deprivation (not needed if already hypernatremic)

Test with exogenous ADH
After 2-4 mcg DDAVP IV or 5 units of vasopressin SQ, a twofold increase in urine osmolality indicates neurogenic/central DI or <10% increase indicates nephrogenic DI

5.3.1   Hypernatremia clinical manifestations

The clinical manifestations of hypernatremia depend upon rapidity of onset, duration, and magnitude of hypernatremia.

Alteration of brain water content with brain volume loss
- **In severe cases:** Substantial brain shrinkage, traction of the venous sinuses and intracerebral veins leading to rupture and hemorrhage
- **In less profound cases:** Nonspecific (nausea, muscle weakness, fasciculations, decreased mental status)

Complications of aggressive treatment
- Adaptation to hypernatremia results in the uptake of "idiogenic osmoles" by brain cells resulting in brain edema when overly rapid rehydration takes place (causing seizures, decreased mental status)

5.3.2   Treatment of hypernatremia

For practical purposes one can imagine that the body maintains the homeostasis of the basic components in the following order of priority:
1. **Circulatory volume**
2. **Osmotic equilibrium**
3. **Electrolyte concentration.**

Similarly, in the treatment of electrolyte disorders, the therapeutic measures should be directed at the same aspects in the same order (eg, attempts to correct the circulatory volume should take priority and precede correction of sodium concentration and osmolality).

Helpful points in treating hypernatremia

- In patients with hypovolemia - start with volume expansion with isotonic saline, then correct water deficit
- In patients with hypervolemia - water + loop diuretic to avoid pulmonary or cerebral edema
- Replace calculated water deficit plus ongoing losses (urinary, GI) plus insensible losses (no more than half of calculated water deficit in the first 24 hours to prevent cerebral edema)
- Reduce Na$^+$ concentration by ≤1 mmol/L/hr if symptomatic initially but <12 mmol/L/day
- When symptoms are resolved, replace the remaining water deficit in 24-48 hours
- Worsening neurologic status after initial improvement suggests brain edema - discontinue water replacement
- Central DI - treat with DDAVP
- Nephrogenic DI: Thiazides: Inhibit urinary diluting capacity and cause mild intravascular volume depletion, which decreases water delivery to the collecting duct, which in turn decreases polyuria for symptomatic benefit
- Amiloride for lithium-induced DI: Like thiazides, amiloride decreases polyuria, but spares K$^+$ wasting and may diminish lithium toxicity (by blocking lithium entry into collecting duct cells in exchange for Na$^+$)

Water deficit to correct in hypernatremia

Water deficit to correct in hypernatremia (assuming distribution volume of Na$^+$ to be 0.6 of the body mass):

$$\text{Water deficit (L)} = \frac{\text{Serum Na (mEq/L)} - 140}{140} \times 0.6 \times \text{Body Mass (Kg)}$$

5.4   Hyponatremia

Hyponatremia is relatively common (1% - 2% of hospitalized patients). Unlike hypernatremia (which is always associated with hypertonicity), hyponatremia can be associated with hypotonicity, isotonicity, or hypertonicity. To identify the cause of hyponatremia one has to collect the following information: Plasma osmolality, patient volume status, urine sodium concentration, and urine osmolality (latter reflects ADH secretion).

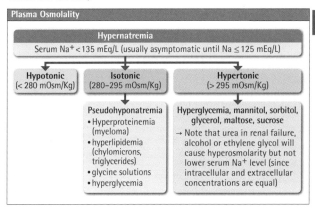

Plasma Osmolality

Hypernatremia

Serum $Na^+ < 135$ mEq/L (usually asymptomatic until Na ≤ 125 mEq/L)

Hypotonic (< 280 mOsm/Kg)

Isotonic (280–295 mOsm/Kg)

Hypertonic (> 295 mOsm/Kg)

Pseudohyponatremia
- Hyperproteinemia (myeloma)
- hyperlipidemia (chylomicrons, triglycerides)
- glycine solutions
- hyperglycemia

Hyperglycemia, mannitol, sorbitol, glycerol, maltose, sucrose
→ Note that urea in renal failure, alcohol or ethylene glycol will cause hyperosmolarity but not lower serum Na^+ level (since intracellular and extracellular concentrations are equal)

Volume Status and Urine Na⁺

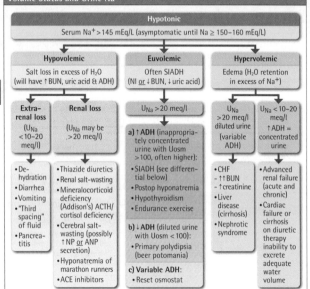

Other helpful points for SIADH:

- Low ADH level results in diluted urine, so that Uosm <100 (eg, in primary poly-dipsia/"beer potomania")
- SIADH is the most common cause of euvolemic hyponatremia
- SIADH is hard to distinguish from cerebral salt wasting as volume status might be difficult to estimate, but cerebral salt wasting is usually due to intracranial hemorrhage. It does not have strict diagnostic criteria or lab tests associated with it, though management is often similar to SIADH.

Hyponatremia   69

Other helpful points (cont.):

- Diagnostic criteria for SIADH: Hypoosmolarity (serum osmolarity <280 mOsm/Kg) hyponatremia (Na$^+$ ≤134 mEq/dL) with clinical euvolemia, urinary Na >40 mEq/dL, inappropriately concentrated urine (U$_{osm}$ >100 mOsm/Kg), normal adrenal, thyroid, cardiac, renal, and hepatic function, frequently with hypouricemia.

Differential Diagnosis of SIADH

SIADH is the most frequent cause of hyponatremia in a hospitalized patient. It is important to identify the underlying cause of SIADH, as it may be due to serious or even urgent medical conditions or may recur

Malignant neoplasia

• Carcinoma (bronchogenic, duodenal, pancreatic, ureteral, prostatic, bladder) • Lymphoma and leukemia	• Thymoma, mesothelioma, and Ewing's sarcoma

CNS disorders

• Trauma, subarachnoid hemorrhage, subdural hematoma • Infection (encephalitis, meningitis, brain abscess)	• Tumors • Porphyria • Stroke • Vasculitis

Pulmonary disorders

• Tuberculosis • Pneumonia • Vasculitis	• Mechanical ventilators with positive pressure • Lung abscess

Drugs

• Desmopressin • Vasopressin • Chlorpropamide • Thiazide diuretics • Oxytocin • Haloperidol	• Phenothiazines • Tricyclic antidepressants • High dose cyclophosphamide • Vincristine • Vinblastine • Nicotine

Others

• "Idiopathic" SIADH • Hypothyroidism • HIV	• Guillain-Barre syndrome • Multiple sclerosis • Nephrogenic SIADH

5.4.1 Clinical manifestations of hyponatremia

Symptoms of hyponatremia depend on:
- Degree and rapidity of onset
- Underlying CNS status and
- Other metabolic factors such as:
  - Hypoxia
  - Acidosis
  - Hypercalcemia
  - Hypercapnia

The underlying mechanism of symptoms is hypoosmolar encephalopathy (brain edema from water shift).
- **Mild symptoms:** Headache, nausea
- **More severe symptoms (usually with Na <125):** Confusion, obtundation, focal neurological deficits, seizures

5.4.2 Treatment of hyponatremia

As in the case of hypernatremia, the therapeutic measures aimed to correct hyponatremia should be directed at correcting the circulatory volume first and only then at correcting the sodium concentration. If the hyponatremia developed rapidly (< 24 h), it should be corrected rapidly; if it developed slowly, it should be corrected slowly to decrease the risk of a CNS demyelinating syndrome.

Treatment of hyponatremia

Euvolemia

Treat if:
- Rapid onset
- Higher degree of hypo-natremia sympto-matic

Hypovolemia

- Start with normal saline (NS), if suspect diuretics ⇒ supplement with K.
- Even if only the potential for hypo-volemia exist (diuretics use, etc.) it is reasonable to give a trial of 1–2 L NS and observe response
- Primary or secondary glucocoticoid deficiency ⇒ glucocorticoid replace-ment after ACTH stimulation test

Hypervolemia

(CHF, liver or kidney disease)
- Start with loop diuretics
- Treat underlying disorder
- Sodium & water restriction
- Inotropes in CHF

Acute Treatment

- Asymptomatic with Na > 120 ⇒ fluid restriction, discontinue any drugs associated with decreased water excretion, salt tablets orally may be used
- If CNS symptoms, use either
  - Hypertonic saline (3% NaCl) ± furosemide (to prevent volume overload in patients with CHF)
  - Normal Saline + loop diuretic (to decrease urine concentrating ability)
- If hyponatremia present over 24h, correct Na at ≤ 0.5 mEq/l/hour. May use desmopressin to slow correction that is occuring too rapidly, if necessary.

Chronic Treatment

- Fluid restriction
- Demeclocycline (600–1200 mg/d) ⇒ causes nephrogenic DI by reversible nephrotoxicity
- Urea or high protein dietary supplementation
- Vasopressin antagonists

Additional considerations for using 3% NaCl

- Stop infusion if symptoms are abolished, or serum Na^+ has risen to ≥125 mEq/L.
- Correct serum Na^+ at 0.5 mEq/L/hour (max 1 mOsm/Kg/h), initially raising Na not more than 8 mEq/L over the first 24 h and 18 mEq/L over the first 48 h.
- Rapid osmolality correction can cause the demyelination syndrome, pontine and extrapontine myelinolysis, with substantial neurological morbidity and mortality.

Calculations to establish the rate of 3% NaCl infusion

Calculations are based on the following assumptions: Although NaCl is distributed mainly in the extracellular space, the distribution volume of NaCl is total body water, or therefore, roughly 0.6 x Body Mass in Kg. The calculations below are crude approximations since they do not account for the rate of Na and water excretion or potassium losses.

As 1 liter of 3% NaCl has 512 mEq of Na^+ (0.512 mEq/ml), if the rate of correction of serum Na^+ is to be 0.5 mEq/L/hour, the rate of infusion of 3% NaCl infusion in ml/hr will be = 0.5/0.512 x 0.6 Body Mass (in Kg)

Calculation of total Na deficit to correct hyponatremia

Calculated **Na Deficit (mEq)** = 0.6 (Body Mass [Kg]) x (140 – Serum Na [mEq/L])

If volume depletion is present, replace estimated volume deficit in liters with normal saline in addition.

Note that the serum Na should usually only be corrected to about 130 mEq/L to avoid overcorrection.

Relative risk vs. benefit in treatment of hyponatremia

	Risk of uncorrected hyponatremia	Risk of demyelination
Rapid onset, symptoms	Higher	Lower
Slow onset, asymptomatic	Lower	Higher

5.5 Hypokalemia

Similar to other electrolytes, hypokalemia can be explained either by lower intake, higher excretion, or intracellular redistribution of potassium. To identify the cause of hypokalemia, the following tests are very helpful: Urine potassium, and for concentrated urines (U_{Osm} >300 mOsm/Kg), the transtubular potassium gradient (TTKG described below), urine chloride, plasma bicarbonate.

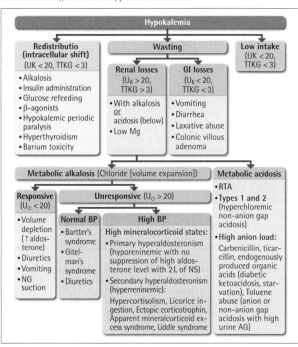

Transtubular K gradient (TTKG)

The concept of TTKG helps to identify renal wasting of potassium (high TTKG), as opposed to GI losses or intracellular shift (low TTKG). TTKG compensates for a high urinary concentration above 300 mOsm/Kg which raises the U_K concentration by removing tubular fluid from the final urine, but without excreting more potassium.

Note that this formula is valid only when U_{Osm} >300 mOsm/Kg and U_{Na} >25 mEq/L and should not be used to "correct" for dilute urines.

$$TTKG = \frac{Urine_K}{Plasma_K} \div \frac{Urine_{Osm}}{Plasma_{Osm}} = \frac{U_K}{P_K} \times \frac{P_{Osm}}{U_{Osm}}$$

> **TTKG < 3**: GI loss, intracellular redistribution with renal K conservation
> **TTKG < 8**: Inadequate renal K excretion when hyperkalemic
> **TTKG > 5**: Renal K wasting when hypokalemic
> **TTKG ≥ 8**: Denotes appropriate aldosterone effect when hyperkalemic

5.5.1   Clinical manifestations of hypokalemia

- ECG changes (prominent U-wave, T wave flattening, ST depression)
- Skeletal muscle weakness to the point of paralysis
- Respiratory arrest may occur with severe hypokalemia
- Decreased motility of the smooth muscle: ileus, urinary retention
- Rhabdomyolysis may occur with severe hypokalemia
- Nephrogenic DI (hypokalemia interferes with concentrating mechanism in the distal nephron)

5.5.2   Treatment of hypokalemia

- Oral or IV K (oral is safer)
- IV (for K <3.0 mEq/L) not more than 10 mmol/h, recheck K every 2-3 h
- Magnitude of K replacement can't be calculated from serum K but is often over 200 mEq when serum K <3.0 mEq/L

5.6   Hyperkalemia

5.6.1   Causes of hyperkalemia

Increased intake
• Use of salt substitutes or K^+ supplements (usually in the setting of CKD)

Redistribution from cells
• Shift of K^+ out of cells due to acidosis, depolarizing paralytic agents (e.g., succinyl choline), or decreased functioning of Na-K-ATPase related to hypoxia, insulin deficiency, beta blockade, or severe digitalis toxicity
• Cell destruction - crush injuries, rhabdomyolysis, burns and hemolysis
• Receiving old or improperly administered blood or massive blood transfusion

Inadequate excretion
• Renal failure
• Hypoaldosteronism or adrenal insufficiency
• Renal tubular defects: Type 4 RTA, interstitial renal diseases
• Medications: aliskiren, ACEI, ARB, aldosterone receptor antagonists , amiloride, trimethoprim, calcineurin inhibitors
• Pseudohypoaldosteronism

5.6.2   Clinical manifestations of hyperkalemia

• Skeletal muscle weakness to the point of paralysis and respiratory failure
• ECG changes

  - Peaking of T-wave   - ST depression
  - 1st degree AV block   - Shallow P-waves → atrial standstill
  - Widening of QRS   - Biphasic waves → ventricular standstill

5.6.3   Acute treatment of hyperkalemia

• Stabilize the myocardium (IV calcium chloride 1 g over 1 minute or calcium gluconate 3 g over 1 min, repeat in 5 min if no ECG improvement)
• Shift K to the intracellular space
  - Insulin at doses of 10 units IV (K decreases in 15-30 min) with glucose (to avoid hypoglycemia)
  - Beta-agonists (K decreases in 30 min): are as effective as insulin for lowering serum potassium and have a longer duration of action but may promote arrhythmia
  - Sodium bicarbonate 50-150 mEq IV (K decreases in 1-4 hours): Supported only by studies with weak and equivocal results but useful when acidotic
• Remove potassium from the body
  - Diuresis
  - Sodium polystyrene sulfonate (Kayexalate) orally or rectally
  - Dialysis

Regulation of Calcium and Phosphate Balance

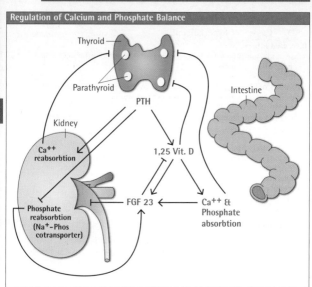

5.7   Hypercalcemia

Causes of Hypercalcemia

Causes of Hypercalcemia

Malignancies (PTH low or normal)	Elevated PTH	Other causes
• Serum parathyroid-related protein (PTHrP): Solid tumors, non-Hodgkin's lymphoma (note that primary or ectopic elevated PTH may co-exist with PTHrP) • 1,25 dihydroxy vitamin D overproduction in Hodgkin's and non-Hodgkin lymphomas • Osteolytic metastatic diseases: Multiple myeloma, breast cancer, some solid tumors (may act through local cytokines and/or PTHrP)	• Primary hyperparathyroidism • Tertiary hyperparathyroidism in advanced CKD	• Endocrine: Hyperthyroidism, adrenal insufficiency • Post-rhabdomyolytic acute renal failure in recovery phase • Familial hypocalciuric hypercalcemia (Ratio of $U_{Ca}/U_{Cr} < 0.1$) • Accelerated bone turnover: Paget's disease with immobilization, prolonged severe immobilization • Granulomatous diseases (1,25 dihydroxy vitamin D overproduction): Tuberculosis, sarcoidosis, fungal diseases, berylliosis • Drugs: Hypervitaminosis of A or D, calcitriol, lithium, thiazides, theophylline toxicity, tamoxifen, milk-alkali syndrome, high calcium intake (particularly with renal disease)

Calcium, phosphate and PTH in hyperparathyroidism, malignancy and vitamin D excess syndromes

	Ca^{++}	Phosphate	PTH
Primary hyperparathyroidism: Adenoma (85%), hyperplasia (15%), or carcinoma (<1%) of the parathyroid glands	↑	↓	↑
Malignancy	↑	↓	↓
1,25 dihydroxy vitamin D overproduction (eg, sarcoidosis)	↑	↑	↓

5.7.1 Clinical manifestations of hypercalcemia

Cardiovascular
- Dysrhythmia
- EKG changes (Short corrected QT interval, broad T waves, 1st degree AV block)
- Digoxin sensitivity
- Hypertension

Gastrointestinal
- Anorexia
- Nausea/vomiting
- Constipation
- Abdominal pain
- Pancreatitis

Genito-urinary
- Polyuria
- Polydipsia
- Nephrolithiasis

Musculo-skeletal
- Muscle weakness
- Hyporeflexia
- Bone Pain
- Fractures

Neurologic
- Insomnia
- Delirium
- Dementia
- Psychosis
- Lethargy
- Somnolence
- Coma

5.7.2 Treatment of hypercalcemia
- Acute treatment if Ca >14 or altered mental status/ECG changes
- Normal saline 2.5-4 L/day + furosemide 10-40 mg IV Q6h
- Calcitonin (Miacalcin)
- Bisphosphonates (pamidronate, zoledronic acid and etidronate)
- Calcimimetics in those with high PTH (cinacalcet)
- Gallium nitrate (Ganite) for cancer-associated hypercalcemia
- Glucocorticoids (especially in hematologic malignancies and sarcoid)
- Estrogens, raloxifene
- Chloroquine for sarcoid
- EDTA (rarely used)
- Dialysis

5.7.3   Indications for parathyroidectomy

Criteria for Parathyroidectomy in Patients With Hyperparathyroidism
In patients with asymptomatic primary hyperparathyroidism
• Serum calcium >1-2 mg/dl (0.25 mmol/l) above the upper limit of the local reference range;   • Creatinine clearance less than 60 ml/min; attributed to calcemic nephropathy   • Age <50 years;   • BMD T-score <-2.5 determined by DXA scan at any site (forearm, lumbar spine, hip)
In secondary/tertiary hyperparathyroidism in ESRD
• Severe hypercalcemia resistant to medical or dialysis treatment   • High total alkaline phosphatase accompanied by specific radiologic and/or his-tomorphologic changes of renal osteopathy   • Hyperphosphatemia resistant to treatment with extraskeletal soft tissue calcifications   • Calciphylaxis   • Symptomatic disease: Pruritus, myopathy   • Marked hyperparathyroidism (PTH level >10 times upper normal limit)

5.8   Hypocalcemia

5.8.1   Clinical manifestations of hypocalcemia

- Muscle spasms, cramps, and tremors
- Hyperactive reflexes
- Diarrhea
- Tingling of the fingers, toes, lips and face
- Tetany
- Positive Trousseau's sign - carpedal spasm (hand spasm when B/P cuff inflated above arterial pressure for 3-4 minutes).
- Positive Chvostek's sign (the twitching of the circumoral muscles with tapping lightly over the facial nerve)
- Seizures
- EKG changes/arrhythmia

5.8.2   Treatment of hypocalcemia

- Monitor lab for other disturbances such as hypokalemia, hyperphosphatemia, hypomagnesemia, and alkalosis
- Cardiac monitor
- Seizure precautions and quiet room to decrease external stimuli
- Administer oral calcium supplements and/or vitamin D for mild to moderate hypocalcemia

Treatment of hypocalcemia (cont.)

- Give oral calcium between meals to increase intestinal absorption
- Administer IV calcium for severe hypocalcemia via slow IV bolus followed by slow IV drip
- Watch for infiltration, calcium chloride can cause necrosis and tissue sloughing. Never give calcium IM or SC.
- Check Chvostek's sign every hour when giving IV calcium.
- Teach patient about foods and fluids high in calcium

5.9   Hypophosphatemia

5.9.1   Causes of hypophosphatemia

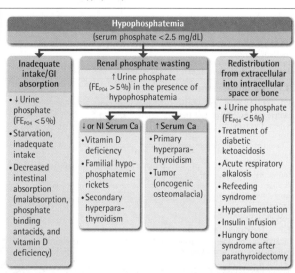

5.10   Hyperphosphatemia

5.10.1   Causes of hyperphosphatemia

Elevated intake	Decreased renal excretion	Redistribution from intracellular to extra-cellular space
• Phosphate containing laxatives or enemas (can cause severe AKI due to phosphate nephropathy)	• Renal failure (Stage >4) • Vitamin D toxicity • Bisphosphonates • Hypoparathyroidism • Acromegaly • Familial tumoral calcinosis	• Rhabdomyolysis • Tumor lysis syndrome • Diabetic ketoacidosis • Lactic acidosis • Severe hemolytic reaction

5.10.2   Treatment of hyperphosphatemia

Treatment is usually undertaken for patients with renal failure to reduce serum phosphate to < 5.5-6.0 mg/dl:
• Dietary phosphate restriction
• Oral phosphate binders to limit intestinal absorption:
  - Calcium carbonate or acetate, usually limited to ≤1.5 gm/d of calcium
  - Sevelamer
  - Lanthanum carbonate
  - Aluminum hydroxide, limit use to short-term AKI to avoid aluminum toxicity
• Dialysis

Fractional excretion of phosphate

Urine phosphate can be either measured in 24 h urine or as a fractional phosphate excretion in a random urine sample:

$$FE_{PO_4} = \frac{\text{(urine phosphate} \times \text{serum creatinine)}}{\text{(serum phosphate} \times \text{urine creatinine)}} \times 100\%$$

FE_{PO4} usually varies between 5% and 20% but may increase to >80% with secondary hyperparathyroidism of renal failure.

5.11   Magnesium: Effects in the Body

Magnesium is fourth most common cation in the body, and the second most common intracellular cation.

• Vasodilatation by direct action on blood vessels (Mg acts as a calcium antagonist) and antisympathetic activity
• Negative inotropic effect
• Bronchodilation
• Tocolytic effect
• Renal vasodilation and diuresis
• Cofactor for many intracellular enzymes
• Responsible for the maintenance of transmembrane gradients of sodium and potassium

Renal Handling of Magnesium

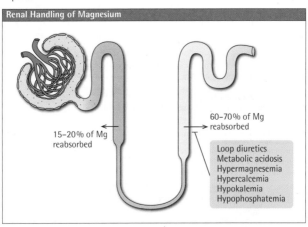

15–20% of Mg reabsorbed

60–70% of Mg reabsorbed

Loop diuretics
Metabolic acidosis
Hypermagnesemia
Hypercalcemia
Hypokalemia
Hypophosphatemia

5.12 Hypomagnesemia

5.12.1 Causes of Hypomagnesemia

- **Low intake or poor GI absorption:**
  - Celiac disease
  - Inflammatory bowel disease
  - Proton pump inhibitors
- **Increased loss**
  - GI loss: Diarrhea, vomiting, laxative use
  - Renal loss: Tubular defect (congenital or acquired), diabetes, alcohol, drugs affecting tubular absorption (diuretics, aminoglycosides, amphotericin, cisplatin, pentamidine, cyclosporine), hypercalcemia
  - Skin loss: excessive sweating
- **Higher requirements**
  - Pregnancy
  - Growth

5.12.2 Clinical manifestations of hypomagnesemia

- Neurological: Nystagmus, convulsions, numbness
- Fatigue
- Muscle spasms, cramps, or muscle weakness
- Cardiac arrhythmias
- Hypocalcemia, hypokalemia
- Cardiac or respiratory arrest, if severe

5.13 Hypermagnesemia

5.13.1 Causes of hypermagnesemia

- Iatrogenic causes, eg, parenteral magnesium
- Excessive use of magnesium-containing laxatives and antacids

5.13.2 Effects of hypermagnesemia

- Depressed central nervous system, muscle weakness
- Depressed cardiac conduction, widened QRS complexes, prolonged P-R interval

5.13.3 Treatment of hypermagnesemia

- Forced diuresis
- Dialysis
- Intravenous calcium

5.14   Magnesium: Therapeutic Use

- Preeclampsia and eclampsia
- Cardiac arrhythmias (torsades de pointes, digoxin toxicity, any serious ventricular or atrial arrhythmies especially also with hypokalemia)
- Asthma
- Refractory hypokalemia in the context of hypomagnesemia

5.15   Polyuria (UO >3000 ml/24h) Workup

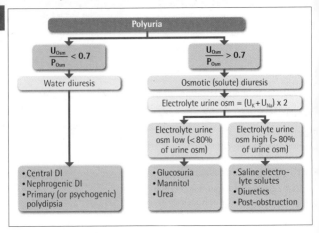

5.16   Diuretic Therapy

	Loop diuretics	Thiazides	Amiloride/ Triamterene
Mechanism	Block Na^+-K^+-Cl^- transporter	Block electro-neutral Na^+-Cl^- transporter	Block apical Na^+ channels
Water and Na^+	Impair urinary concentration ability: Water is excreted in excess of sodium	Impair the ability to dilute urine and excrete a water load while diuresing sodium	
Other electrolytes	Loss of K^+ and Mg^{++}, increased urinary Ca^{++} excretion	Loss of K^+ and Mg^{++}, urinary Ca^{++} retention	Impair the excretion of K^+ and H^+ in exchange for Na^+ absorption

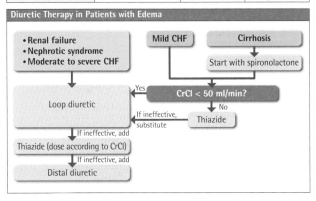

Diuretic Therapy in Patients with Edema

References and Suggested Reading

Sodium

Adrogué HJ, Madias NE. The challenge of hyponatremia. J Am Soc Nephrol. 2012; 23(7):1140–8.

Verbalis JG, Goldsmith SR, Greenberg A, et al. Hyponatremia treatment guidelines 2007: Expert panel recommendations. Am J Med 2007: 120(11 Suppl 1):S1-21.

Hannon MJ, Thompson CJ. The syndrome of inappropriate antidiuretic hormone: prevalence, causes and consequences. Eur J Endocrinol,2010; 162(6): Suppl 1 S5-12.

Sterns RH, Nigwekar SU, Hix JK. The treatment of hyponatremia. Semin Nephrol 2009; 29(3):282-99.

Sterns RH, Hix JK, Silver S. Treatment of hyponatremia. Curr Opin Nephrol Hypertens 2010; 19(5):493-8.

Sterns RH, Silver SM. Cerebral salt wasting versus SIADH: what difference? J Am Soc Nephrol. 2008;19(2):194-196.

Hix JK, Silver S, Sterns RH. Diuretic-associated hyponatremia. Semin Nephrol 2011; 31(6):553-66.

Glover M, Clayton J. Thiazide-induced hyponatraemia: epidemiology and clues to pathogenesis. Cardiovasc Ther 2012; 30(5):e219-26.

Lien YH, Shapiro JI, Chan L. Effects of hypernatremia on organic brain osmoles. J Clin Invest. 1990;85(5):1427-1435.

Noakes TD. Overconsumption of fluids by athletes. BMJ. 2003;327(7407):113-114.

Offenstadt G, Das V. Hyponatremia, hypernatremia: a physiological approach. Minerva Anestesiol, 2006; 72(6):353-6.

Feldman BJ, Rosenthal SM, Vargas GA, et al. Nephrogenic syndrome of inappropriate antidiuresis. N Engl J Med 2005; 352(18):1884-90.

Potassium

Harel Z, Gilbert C, Wald R, et al. The effect of combination treatment with aliskiren and blockers of the renin-angiotensin system on hyperkalaemia and acute kidney injury: systematic review and meta-analysis. BMJ. 2012;344:e42.

Khan FY. Rhabdomyolysis: a review of the literature. Neth J Med. 2009;67(9):272-283.

Elliott MJ, Ronksley PE, Clase CM, Ahmed SB, Hemmelgarn BR. Management of patients with acute hyperkalemia. CMAJ. 2010;182(15):1631-1635.

Lin SH, Lin YF, Chen DT, et al. Laboratory tests to determine the cause of hypokalemia and paralysis. Arch Intern Med,2004; 164:1561-6.

Nappi JM, Sieg A. Aldosterone and aldosterone receptor antagonists in patients with chronic heart failure. Vasc Health Risk Manag. 2011;7:353-363.

Sihler KC, Napolitano LM. Complications of massive transfusion. Chest. 2010;137(1):209-220.

Calcium

Makras P, Papapoulos SE. Medical treatment of hypercalcaemia. Hormones (Athens), 2009; 8:83-95.

Peacock M. Calcium metabolism in health and disease. Clin J Am Soc Nephrol. 2010;5 Suppl 1:S23-30.

Schlosser K, Zielke A, Rothmund M. Medical and surgical treatment for secondary and tertiary hyperparathyroidism. Scand J Surg. 2004;93(4):288-297.

Varghese J, Rich T, Jimenez C. Benign familial hypocalciuric hypercalcemia. Endocr Pract. 2011;17 Suppl 1:13-17.

Khan A, Grey A, Shoback D. Medical management of asymptomatic primary hyperparathyroidism: proceedings of the third international workshop. J Clin Endocrinol Metab. 2009;94(2):373-381.

References and Suggested Reading (cont.)

Chitambar CR. Medical applications and toxicities of gallium compounds. Int J Environ Res Public Health. 2010;7(5):2337-2361.

Grieff M, Bushinsky DA. Diuretics and disorders of calcium homeostasis. Semin Nephrol 2011; 31(6): 535-41.

Phosphate

Gaasbeek A, Meinders AE. Hypophosphatemia: an update on its etiology and treatment. Am J Med 2005; 118(10):1094-101.

Assadi F. Hypophosphatemia: an evidence-based problem-solving approach to clinical cases. Iran J Kidney Dis, 2010; 4: 195-201.

Subramanian R, Khardori R. Severe hypophosphatemia. Pathophysiologic implications,clinical presentations, and treatment. Medicine (Baltimore) 2000; 79(1):1-8.

Liamis G, Milionis HJ, Elisaf M. Medication-induced hypophosphatemia: a review. QJM 2010; 103(7): 449-59.

Delmez JA, Slatopolsky E. Hyperphosphatemia: its consequences and treatment in patients with chronic renal disease. Am J Kidney Dis. 1992; 19(4):303-17.

Friedman EA. Consequences and management of hyperphosphatemia in patients with renal insufficiency. Kidney Int Suppl. 2005; Jun (95):S1-7.

Levin A, Bakris GL, Molitch M, et al. Prevalence of abnormal serum vitamin D, PTH, calcium, and phosphorus in patients with chronic kidney disease: results of the study to evaluate early kidney disease. Kidney Int. 2007; 71(1):31-8.

Wahl P, Wolf M. FGF23 in chronic kidney disease. Adv Exp Med Biol. 2012;728:107-25.

KDIGO 2012 Clinical Practice Guideline for the Evaluation and Management of Chronic Kidney Disease. Chap 3: Management of progression and complications of CKD. Kidney International Supplements (2013) 3, 73-90

Magnesium

Byrd RP, Jr, Roy TM. Magnesium: its proven and potential clinical significance. South Med J. 2003;96(1):104.

Fawcett WJ, Haxby EJ, Male DA. Magnesium: physiology and pharmacology. Br J Anaesth. 1999;83(2):302-320.

Fox C, Ramsoomair D, Carter C. Magnesium: its proven and potential clinical significance. South Med J. 2001;94(12):1195-1201.

Quamme GA. Renal magnesium handling: new insights in understanding old problems. Kidney Int. 1997;52(5):1180-1195.

Saris NE, Mervaala E, Karppanen H, et al. Magnesium. An update on physiological, clinical and analytical aspects. Clin Chim Acta. 2000;294(1-2):1-26

Polyuria

Christensen JH, Rittig S. Familial neurohypophyseal diabetes insipidus--an update. Semin Nephrol. 2006; 26(3):209-23.

Smoyer WE. Medical management of postobstructive polyuria. Am J Dis Child. 1991; 145(12):1345-8

References and Suggested Reading (cont.)

Diuretics

Wile D. Diuretics: a review. Ann Clin Biochem 2012; 49(Pt 5):419-31.

Sica DA, Carter B, Cushman W, Hamm L. Thiazide and loop diuretics. J Clin Hypertens (Greenwich) 2011; 13(9):639-43.

Kassamali R, Sica DA. Acetazolamide: a forgotten diuretic agent. Cardiol Rev 2011; 19(6):276-8.

Epstein M, Calhoun DA. Aldosterone blockers (mineralocorticoid receptor antagonism) and potassium-sparing diuretics. J Clin Hypertens (Greenwich) 2011; 13(9):644-8

Ernst ME, Gordon JA. Diuretic therapy: key aspects in hypertension and renal disease. J Nephrol 2010; 23(5):487-93.

Sarafidis PA, Georgianos PI, Lasaridis AN. Diuretics in clinical practice. Part I: mechanisms of action, pharmacological effects and clinical indications of diuretic compounds. Expert Opin Drug Saf 2010; 9(2):243-57.

Sarafidis PA, Georgianos PI, Lasaridis AN. Diuretics in clinical practice. Part II: electrolyte and acid-base disorders complicating diuretic therapy. Expert Opin Drug Saf 2010; 9(2):259-73.

Palmer BF. Metabolic complications associated with use of diuretics. Semin Nephrol 2011; 31(6):542-52.

Brater DC. Update in diuretic therapy: clinical pharmacology. Semin Nephrol 2011; 31(6):483-94.

Bernstein PL, Ellison DH. Diuretics and salt transport along the nephron. Semin Nephrol 2011; 31(6):475-82.

6   Acid-base Disorders

6.1   Introduction

This chapter discusses how to use arterial or venous blood gas results and routine serum electrolytes to identify an acid-base disorder.

Henderson-Hasselbalch equation

Interpretations of blood gas findings start with the Henderson-Hasselbalch equation:

$$\textbf{pH} = pK_a + \log \frac{[\text{Base}]}{[\text{Acid}]} \quad \text{where } pK_a \text{ is the negative log of the acid dissociation constant}$$

The blood buffering system uses bicarbonate as the base and carbonic acid as the acid; therefore this equation can be rewritten as follows:

$$\textbf{pH} = pK_a + \log \frac{[HCO_3]}{[H_2CO_3]}$$

Using a pKa value of 6.1 for carbonic acid, and a conversion factor of 0.03 to express the acid concentration in terms of partial arterial pressure of CO_2 (p_aCO_2), which is measured in arterial blood gases (ABGs), this is finally rewritten as follows:

$$\textbf{pH} = 6.1 + \log \frac{[HCO_3]}{0.03p_aCO_2}$$

Since this final expression includes a logarithm, which is difficult for quick bedside calculation, several simple approximations may be used, as discussed on the pages that follow.

Note that a normal pH of 7.4, the concentration of the base $[HCO_3]$ of about 25 mEq/L is 20 times that of carbonic acid with a concentration of 1.2 mEq/L (or a pCO_2 of 40 mm Hg).

6.2   Acid-base Disorder Diagnostic Algorithm

This algorithm provides an interpretation of ABGs in conjunction with plasma chemistry.

To use this algorithm:
• First examine the pH and identify acidemia or alkalemia.
• Then, using the bicarbonate (HCO_3) concentration obtained from serum electrolytes and the $paCO_2$ from the ABG, identify whether the primary cause of the disorder is metabolic or respiratory (see ABG algorithm below)
• Then perform a calculation to examine whether a primary respiratory disorder has appropriate metabolic compensation, or a primary metabolic disorder has appropriate respiratory compensation (refer to the "Compensation" table on the next page)
• If not, there is a second primary disorder, considered to be a "complex" (meaning more than just one) acid-base disorder, rather than a "simple" (meaning a single) acid-base disorder underlying the observed changes

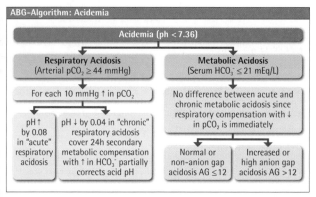

ABG-Algorithm: Acidemia

Acidemia (ph < 7.36)

Respiratory Acidosis
(Arterial pCO₂ ≥ 44 mmHg)

Metabolic Acidosis
(Serum HCO₃⁻ ≤ 21 mEq/L)

For each 10 mmHg ↑ in pCO₂

No difference between acute and chronic metabolic acidosis since respiratory compensation with ↓ in pCO₂ is immediately

pH ↑ by 0.08 in "acute" respiratory acidosis

pH ↓ by 0.04 in "chronic" respiratory acidosis cover 24h secondary metabolic compensation with ↑ in HCO₃⁻ partially corrects acid pH

Normal or non-anion gap acidosis AG ≤12

Increased or high anion gap acidosis AG >12

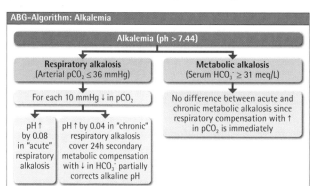

ABG-Algorithm: Alkalemia

Alkalemia (ph > 7.44)

Respiratory alkalosis
(Arterial $pCO_2 \leq 36$ mmHg)

Metabolic alkalosis
(Serum $HCO_3^- \geq 31$ meq/L)

For each 10 mmHg ↓ in pCO_2

pH ↑ by 0.08 in "acute" respiratory alkalosis

pH ↑ by 0.04 in "chronic" respiratory alkalosis cover 24h secondary metabolic compensation with ↓ in HCO_3^- partially corrects alkaline pH

No difference between acute and chronic metabolic alkalosis since respiratory compensation with ↑ in pCO_2 is immediately

Compensation for Respiratory Alkalosis	Compensation for Respiratory Acidosis
Acute	**Acute**
When acute, expect serum HCO_3 to fall about 2 mEq/L for each 10 mm Hg decrease in pCO_2 for normal metabolic compensation	When acute, expect serum HCO_3 to rise about 1 mEq/L for each 10 mm Hg increase in pCO2 for normal metabolic compensation
Chronic	**Chronic**
When over 24 hours, expect serum HCO_3 to fall about 5 mEq/L for each 10 mmHg decrease in pCO_2 for normal metabolic compensation	When over 24 hours, expect serum HCO_3 to rise about 3.5 mEq/L for each 10 mmHg increase in pCO_2 for normal metabolic compensation

Compensation for Metabolic Alkalosis	Compensation for Metabolic Acidosis
There are 3 common ways to evaluate for normal respiratory compensation response (±2 mmHg): • Expect pCO_2 to rise 0.7 mmHg for each 1 mEq/L rise in serum HCO_3^- for normal respiratory compensation • pCO_2 should be equal to serum HCO_3 + 15 mm Hg up to a pCO_2 of about 60 when the pCO_2 rises no further • The easy way: pCO_2 should be equal to the last 2 digits of the pH up to pH 7.60	There are 3 common ways to evaluate for normal respiratory compensation response (±2 mmHg): • Expect pCO_2 to decrease 1.2 mmHg for each 1 mEq/L fall in HCO_3 • pCO_2 should be = 1.5 (HCO_3) + 8 • The easy way: pCO_2 should be equal to the last 2 digits of the pH down to pH 7.10

Useful tips

• Acid-base disorders do not compensate completely, so if the pH is acidic, assume acidosis, if it's alkaline, assume alkalosis.
• In interpreting serum bicarbonate level:
  - If HCO_3 is ↑, there is either a primary metabolic alkalosis or compensation for a respiratory acidosis
  - If HCO_3 is ↓, there is either a primary metabolic acidosis or compensation for a respiratory alkalosis
• If HCO_3 is normal, there is either a normal acid-base state or a complex (double or triple) disorder may be present
• An ↑anion gap almost always indicates a metabolic acidosis
• Serum K^+ concentration may be helpful: If K^+ is ↓, there is usually an alkalosis, if K is ↑, there is usually an acidosis
• When BUN and creatinine levels are ↑, renal failure may be associated with a metabolic acidosis that often has a normal anion gap when mild, and an increased anion gap when renal failure is more severe
• Liver failure is usually associated with metabolic acidosis

6.3   Metabolic Acidosis

6.3.1   Causes of metabolic acidosis

- Once the diagnosis of metabolic acidosis is established, the next step is to identify the cause
- The first step is to assess whether the metabolic acidosis is associated with a normal anion gap or an abnormally high anion gap as shown on the algorithm below
- An increased anion gap indicates the presence of unmeasured acids which may be endogenous, eg, lactic acid, or exogenous, eg, oxalic acid from ethylene glycol poisoning.
- Metabolic acidosis with a normal anion gap is caused by either loss of bicarbonate (from the GI tract or in the urine) or failure to excrete acid [H^+] by the kidneys.

6.3.2   Serum osmolar gap

Using the serum or plasma osmolar gap will help to differentiate between a non-osmolar gap (usually endogenous) and a high osmolar gap (exogenous toxin) acidosis. The osmolar gap is determined by comparing the measured serum or plasma osmolality to the calculated serum osmolality

Serum osmolality

Calculated serum osmolality (to compare with measured S_{Osm} for assessment of an osmolar gap):

$$S_{Osm} = 2\,(Na^+) + \frac{Glucose\ (mg/dL)}{18} + \frac{BUN\ (mg/dL)}{2.8}$$

Metabolic Acidosis: Anion Gap

Metabolic Acidosis

Calculate: Anion gap = $(Na^+) - (HCO_3^- + Cl^-)$

Normal anion gap (10 ± 2):
Hyperchloremic acidosis (loss of bicarbonate with increased renal tubular reabsorption of Cl^-)

Increased anion gap (>12)
Addition of an "unmeasured" acid

Non-anion gap mnemonic: DR. DOOFUS

D – Diarrhea: GI loss of HCO_3^- (expect low urine Na)
R – Renal tubular acidosis (RTA)

D – Drugs: Acetazolamide or topiramate can cause urinary HCO_3^- wasting; tenofovir or ifosfamide can cause RTA
O – Obstructive uropathy
O – Other: Recovery from hyperventilation (the pCO_2 rises, but the HCO_3^- may remain low longer), rapid dilution by intravenous saline can dilute serum HCO_3
F – Fistula: Ileal conduit for bladder replacement or uretero-colonic fistula
U – Uremia in early stages may have non-anion gap acidosis
S – Sniffing glue (toluene poisoning, which may also have an increased anion gap)

Anion gap mnemonic: DR. MAPLES

D – Diabetic ketoacidosis
R – Renal failure

M – Methanol
A – Aspirin
P – Paraldehyde; propylene glycol
L – Lactic acid
E – Ethylene glycol; ethanol ketoacidosis
S – Starvation ketoacidosis

6.3.3   Non-anion gap metabolic acidosis

Renal tubular acidosis (RTA) vs gastrointestinal losses

In metabolic acidosis associated with a normal anion gap, the low serum bicarbonate is either due to loss of bicarbonate from the GI tract from diarrhea, or from failure of the kidneys to conserve bicarbonate or to regenerate bicarbonate by excreting acid. The differential diagnosis between these two conditions is based on showing a normal renal response to acidemia in GI losses. First, the urine pH should be acidic. Second, the urine anion gap should be negative, indicating the presence of the unmeasured urinary cation, NH_4^+, which provides additional acid excretion. If renal tubular NH_4^+ secretion is impaired, the urinary anion gap remains positive or around zero. Remember that calculating a urine anion gap has no role in an increased anion gap metabolic acidosis because there is an unmeasured anion in the urine that obscures the quantity of the unmeasured NH_4^+ cation.

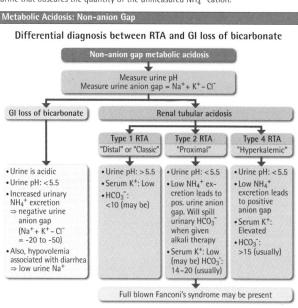

Metabolic Acidosis: Non-anion Gap

Differential diagnosis between RTA and GI loss of bicarbonate

Non-anion gap metabolic acidosis

Measure urine pH
Measure urine anion gap = $Na^+ + K^+ - Cl^-$

GI loss of bicarbonate

Renal tubular acidosis

| Type 1 RTA "Distal" or "Classic" | Type 2 RTA "Proximal" | Type 4 RTA "Hyperkalemic" |

GI loss of bicarbonate:
- Urine is acidic
- Urine pH: < 5.5
- Increased urinary NH_4^+ excretion ⇒ negative urine anion gap ($Na^+ + K^+ - Cl^-$ = -20 to -50)
- Also, hypovolemia associated with diarrhea ⇒ low urine Na^+

Type 1 RTA:
- Urine pH: > 5.5
- Serum K^+: Low
- HCO_3^-: < 10 (may be)

Type 2 RTA:
- Urine pH: < 5.5
- Low NH_4^+ excretion leads to pos. urine anion gap. Will spill urinary HCO_3^- when given alkali therapy
- Serum K^+: Low (may be) HCO_3^-: 14–20 (usually)

Type 4 RTA:
- Urine pH: < 5.5
- Low NH_4^+ excretion leads to positive anion gap
- Serum K^+: Elevated
- HCO_3^-: > 15 (usually)

Full blown Fanconi's syndrome may be present

6.3.4   Types of renal tubular acidosis

The patterns of renal tubular acidosis of Types 1, 2, and 4 are described below. Type 3, renal tubular acidosis, (a mixture of Types 1 and 2), was associated with renal insufficiency and is no longer recognized. Localization of the defect in the nephron is illustrated on the following page.

Distal (Type 1)	Proximal (Type 2)	Hyperkalemic (Type 4)
Features		
• Selective deficit of H^+ secretion in the distal nephron with increased K^+ secretion $\Rightarrow$ alkalotic urine with hyperchloremia and hypokalemia. • May often be associated with secondary hypercalciuria, hypocitraturia and nephrolithiasis	• Inability to reabsorb filtered HCO_3^- with bicarbonate wasting (e.g. carbonic anhydrase inhibitors) $\Rightarrow$ hyperchloremia, normal or low serum K^+, acidic urine: pH <5.5 once serum bicarbonate is low • Not associated with nephrolithiasis except when carbonic anhydrase inhibitors cause proximal tubular HCO_3^- wasting	• Is often called hyporeninemic hypoaldosteronism (though often renin level is not low). • ↓ Aldosterone $\Rightarrow$ impaired renal tubular Na^+ reabsorption leading to impaired K^+ and H^+ secretion with impaired ability to generate $NH_3^- \Rightarrow NH_4^+$ excretion $\Rightarrow$ hyperchloremia, hyperkalemia, acidic urine • Can also be caused by tubulointerstitial renal diseases, eg, lupus nephritis, causing unresponsiveness to aldosterone
Underlying causes		
• Familial • Toluene toxicity • Sjögren's syndrome • Rheumatoid arthritis • Active cirrhosis. • Obstructive uropathy and SLE may cause Type1 RTA with hyperkalemia	• Multiple myeloma with light chain nephropathy • Heavy metals • Tenofovir • Ifosfamide • Hereditary in children	• Diabetic or hypertensive nephropathy (usually with hypoaldosteronism) • Tubulointerstitial diseases • Potassium-sparing diuretics, ACE inhibitors, ARBs, and trimethoprim cause drug-induced Type 4 RTA

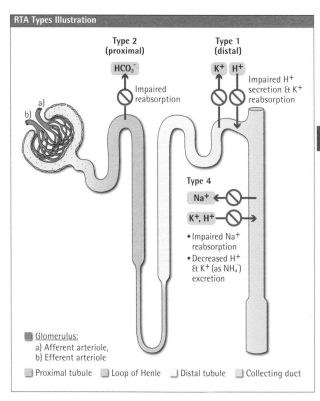

RTA Types Illustration

6.3.5 Types of lactic acidosis

Lactic acidosis is one of the most common types of metabolic acidosis associated with an increased anion gap. The diagram below illustrates underlying causes of lactic acidosis of type A (caused by tissue hypoxia) and type B (associated with other causes of increased lactate generation or decreased excretion).

Lactic Acidosis	
Type A	**Type B**
Tissue hypoxia • Circulatory insufficiency (shock, heart failure) • Severe anemia • Cholera • Mitochondrial enzyme defects and inhibitors (CO, cyanide) • Tumor lysis syndrome	Lactate overproduction and/or decreased hepatic removal of lactate • Hypoglycemia (glycogen storage disease) • Seizures • Diabetes mellitus • Ethanol • Hepatic failure • Malignancy • Medications: Carboplatin, antiretrovirals , salicylates, metformin • Thiamine deficiency (cofactor in oxidative phosphorylation) • D-lactic acidosis

Treatment of lactic acidosis

• Treat underlying condition (eg, restore tissue perfusion)
• Avoid vasoconstrictors but need caution to avoid fluid overload from volume expansion
• Bicarbonate therapy for pH <7.1 (be aware that bicarbonate stimulates phosphofructokinase $\Rightarrow$ leading to enhanced lactate production, can increase pCO_2, and cause overshoot alkalosis after lactate converts to bicarbonate)

Alkalinizing Therapy

Alkalinizing therapy for severe acidemia, of which sodium bicarbonate is the most commonly used agent should be considered in non-anion-gap metabolic acidosis and when pH is <7.1.

Bicarbonate administration guidelines

- Goal - return pH to ≥7.2 and serum bicarbonate to >8-10 (goal is pH 7.45-7.5 in case of salicylate poisoning to enhance excretion)
- Calculate bicarbonate deficit initially using a distribution volume of bicarbonate of 0.5 x body weight in Kg. This is an approximation due to the need to alkalinize both HCO_3^- and other buffers
- Administer sodium bicarbonate as infusion rather than boluses which can be used in severe acidemia
- Check bicarbonate level after ≥30 min has elapsed after infusion is completed.

Potential complications of bicarbonate therapy

- Fluid overload
- Alkalemia occurring as post recovery respiratory alkalosis or as "overshoot" metabolic alkalosis (in lactic acidosis, when lactate is converted to bicarbonate)
- Hypernatremia, hyperosmolality
- May promote precipitation of Ca phosphate and can induce or exacerbate hypocalcemia
- May increase pCO_2 with paradoxical worsening of intracellular acidosis

Alternative alkalinizing agents to $NaHCO_3$

Carbicarb - Na bicarbonate + Na carbonate
- Limits generation of CO_2
- Minimal ↑ in pCO_2

THAM: 0.3N tromethamine - buffers metabolic and respiratory acids (but rarely used):
Reactions take place as follows: Since THAM is a proton acceptor
$(THAM + H^+ \rightarrow THAM^+)$, carbonic acid is buffered as follows:
$THAM + H_2CO_3 \rightarrow THAM^+ + HCO_3^-$
- Limits CO_2 generation
- Side effects: Hyperkalemia, hypoglycemia, ventilatory depression, local injury in cases of extravasation, hepatic necrosis in neonates

6.4   Metabolic Alkalosis

6.4.1   Causes of metabolic alkalosis

Metabolic alkalosis is caused by H^+ and Cl^- loss, or bicarbonate accumulation

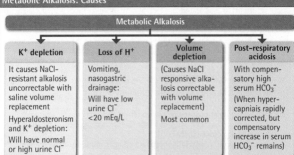

Metabolic Alkalosis: Causes

Metabolic Alkalosis

K⁺ depletion

It causes NaCl-resistant alkalosis uncorrectable with saline volume replacement

Hyperaldosteronism and K^+ depletion: Will have normal or high urine Cl^-

Loss of H⁺

Vomiting, nasogastric drainage: Will have low urine Cl^- <20 mEq/L

Volume depletion

(Causes NaCl responsive alkalosis correctable with volume replacement)

Most common

Post-respiratory acidosis

With compensatory high serum HCO_3^-

(When hypercapnia is rapidly corrected, but compensatory increase in serum HCO_3^- remains)

Mechanism

1. Na^+ reabsorbed in renal tubule in exchange for H^+ rather than K^+ which is depleted leads to loss of H^+ - acidic urine
2. K^+ moves out of cells in exchange or H^+ which in turn moves into the cells

Mechanism

1. Increased tubular reabsorption of Na^+ and HCO_3^- and secretion of H^+ in exchange for Na^+ - leads to rise serum HCO_3^-
2. "Contraction of volume" around HCO_3^- due to low Cl^- from loss of HCl, NaCl, or KCl
3. Leads to increased tubular reabsorption of Cl^- (low urine Cl^- <20 mEq/L is a measure of volume depletion)

6.4.2 Diagnostic workup

Diagnostic workup into causes of metabolic alkalosis is based on the following tests: urine chloride and potassium concentrations and arterial blood pressure.
The figure below shows an algorithm of the workup process

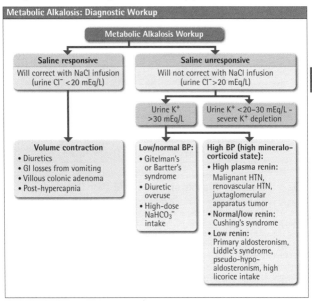

Metabolic Alkalosis: Diagnostic Workup

Metabolic Alkalosis Workup

Saline responsive
Will correct with NaCl infusion
(urine Cl^- < 20 mEq/L)

Saline unresponsive
Will not correct with NaCl infusion
(urine Cl^- > 20 mEq/L)

Urine K^+ > 30 mEq/L

Urine K^+ < 20–30 mEq/L - severe K^+ depletion

Volume contraction
• Diuretics
• GI losses from vomiting
• Villous colonic adenoma
• Post-hypercapnia

Low/normal BP:
• Gitelman's or Bartter's syndrome
• Diuretic overuse
• High-dose $NaHCO_3^-$ intake

High BP (high mineralo-corticoid state):
• **High plasma renin:** Malignant HTN, renovascular HTN, juxtaglomerular apparatus tumor
• **Normal/low renin:** Cushing's syndrome
• **Low renin:** Primary aldosteronism, Liddle's syndrome, pseudo-hypo-aldosteronism, high licorice intake

6.4.3   Treatment of metabolic alkalosis

- Saline for NaCl responsive metabolic alkalosis due to volume depletion or GI losses
- Potassium chloride for K^+ and Cl^- depletion in saline-resistant metabolic alkalosis
- Acetazolamide to lower high serum bicarbonate post-hypercapnia or when hypervolemic
- HCl 0.3N rarely used (needs central intravenous catheter infusion)

Potassium and Acid-base Balance Interrelation

The diagram below illustrates the association between alkalosis and hypokalemia and between acidosis and hyperkalemia

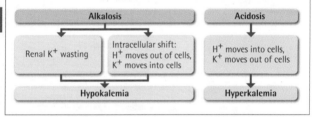

6.5   "Complex" (Double or Triple) Acid-base Disorders

A single patient may have two or even three primary acid-base disorders. It is possible to have a primary metabolic acidosis, eg, diabetic ketoacidosis, and a simultaneous primary metabolic alkalosis, eg, vomiting with HCl loss. This can be diagnosed using the anion gap. In an increased anion gap metabolic acidosis, a "hidden" metabolic alkalosis can be discovered with the "delta/delta" concept. It is based on the assumption that for a given increase in the anion gap (Δ AG), there is a concomitant decrease in bicarbonate concentration (Δ HCO_3) from the added unmeasured acid titrating away the bicarbonate.

The Delta/Delta calculation:

Δ **AG**   = Measured AG – Normal AG (12 mEq/L)   = Unmeasured anions

Δ **HCO$_3$** = Normal HCO$_3$ (24 mEq/L) – measured HCO$_3$ = Fall in HCO$_3$

If Δ AG/Δ HCO$_3$ >2 it suggests a concomitant metabolic alkalosis.

Looked at another way, if the unmeasured anions in the large anion gap were rapidly metabolized to HCO$_3$, the patient would have a high serum bicarbonate level and become alkalotic. This would indicate the concomitance of both a metabolic acidosis and alkalosis. Were such a patient to also overbreathe or underbreathe, the added primary respiratory disorder would give rise to a triple acid-base disturbance.

It is important to note that because there are other buffers besides serum bicarbonate, the AG often increases somewhat more than the serum bicarbonate falls, so the Δ AG/Δ HCO$_3$ is usually >1; between 1 and 2 is usual, in a simple increased anion gap metabolic acidosis.

However, if the AG is significantly less than the fall in serum bicarbonate, it suggests that there may be a concomitant primary non-anion gap metabolic acidosis from loss of HCO$_3$, eg, from diarrhea. This can be calculated as follows: Δ AG/Δ HCO$_3$ <1 suggests a combined normal (non-anion) and high anion gap metabolic acidosis.

References and Suggested Reading

Acid base balance and analysis

Koeppen BM. The kidney and acid-base regulation. Adv Physiol Educ (2009 Dec) 33(4):275-81.

Narins RG Emmett M. Simple and mixed acid-base disorders: a practical approach. Medicine (Baltimore) (1980 May) 59(3):161-8.

Adrogue HJ Madias NE. Secondary responses to altered acid-base status: the rules of engagement. J Am Soc Nephrol (2010 Jun) 21(6):920-3.

Wiederseiner JM Muser J Lutz T Hulter HN Krapf R. Acute metabolic acidosis: characterization and diagnosis of the disorder and the plasma potassium response. J Am Soc Nephrol (2004 Jun) 15(6):1589-96

Bushinsky DA Coe FL Katzenberg C Szidon JP Parks JH. Arterial PCO2 in chronic metabolic acidosis. Kidney Int (1982 Sep) 22(3):311-4.

Krapf R Beeler I Hertner D Hulter HN. Chronic respiratory alkalosis. The effect of sustained hyperventilation on renal regulation of acid-base equilibrium. N Engl J Med (1991 May 16) 324(20):1394-401

Fulop M. A guide for predicting arterial CO2 tension in metabolic acidosis. Am J Nephrol (1997) 17(5):421-4

Rastegar A. Clinical utility of Stewart's method in diagnosis and management of acid-base disorders. Clin J Am Soc Nephrol (2009 Jul) 4(7):1267-74.

Kurtz I, Kraut J, Ornekian V, Nguyen MK. Acid-base analysis: a critique of the Stewart and bicarbonate-centered approaches. Am J Physiol Renal Physiol (2008 May) 294(5):F1009-31.

Anion gap in metabolic acidosis

Reddy P, Mooradian AD. Clinical utility of anion gap in deciphering acid-base disorders. Int J Clin Pract (2009 Oct) 63(10):1516-25

Emmett M Narins RG. Clinical use of the anion gap. Medicine (Baltimore) (1977 Jan) 56(1):38-54

Yan MT, Chau T, Cheng CJ, Lin SH. Hunting down a double gap metabolic acidosis. Ann Clin Biochem. 2010 May;47(Pt 3):267-70.

Fidkowski C, Helstrom J. Diagnosing metabolic acidosis in the critically ill: bridging the anion gap, Stewart, and base excess methods. Can J Anaesth (2009 Mar) 56(3):247-56.

Clinical Acid Base Disorders

Carmody JB, Norwood VF. A clinical approach to paediatric acid-base disorders. Postgrad Med J (2012 Mar) 88(1037):143-51

Dzierba AL, Abraham P. A practical approach to understanding acid-base abnormalities in critical illness. J Pharm Pract (2011 Feb) 24(1):17-26.

Bruno CM, Valenti M. Acid-base disorders in patients with chronic obstructive pulmonary disease: a pathophysiological review. J Biomed Biotechnol (2012) 2012:915150.

Kelly AM. Review article: Can venous blood gas analysis replace arterial in emergency medical care. Emerg Med Australas (2010 Dec) 22(6):493-8.

Malatesha G, Singh NK, Bharija A, et al. Comparison of arterial and venous pH, bicarbonate, PCO2 and PO2 in initial emergency department assessment. Emerg Med J (2007 Aug) 24(8):569-71.

Scale T, Harvey JN. Diabetes, metformin and lactic acidosis. Clin Endocrinol (Oxf). 2011 Feb;74(2):191-6.

Lalau JD, Lacroix C, Compagnon P, et al. Role of metformin accumulation in metformin-associated lactic acidosis. Diabetes Care. 1995 Jun;18(6):779-84.

Ruiz JP, Singh AK, Hart P. Type B lactic acidosis secondary to malignancy: case report, review of published cases, insights into pathogenesis, and prospects for therapy. ScientificWorldJournal. 2011;11:1316-24.

References and Suggested Reading (cont.)

Brivet FG, Slama A, Prat D, Jacobs FM. Carboplatin: a new cause of severe type B lactic acidosis secondary to mitochondrial DNA damage. Am J Emerg Med. 2011 Sep;29(7):842 e5-7.

Goldfarb-Rumyantzev AS, Jeyakumar A, Gumpeni R, Rubin D. Lactic acidosis associated with nucleoside analog therapy in an HIV-positive patient. AIDS Patient Care STDS. 2000 Jul;14(7):339-42.

Hoste EA, Colpaert K, Vanholder RC, et al. Sodium bicarbonate versus THAM in ICU patients with mild metabolic acidosis. J Nephrol. 2005 May-Jun;18(3):303-7.

7 Glomerular Diseases

Glomerular disease may present either with a nephritic pattern (proliferative, inflammatory histology) or a nephrotic pattern (nonproliferative or fibrotic/sclerotic histology) or both together. The initial presentation is very helpful in establishing an initial differential diagnosis.

Nephrotic	Nephritic
• Proteinuria ≥3g/24h/1.73m^2 • Lipiduria (free fat, fatty casts, oval fat bodies) • Hypoalbuminemia • Hyperlipidemia • Edema is common • May be complicated by thrombosis, infection, atherosclerosis, malnutrition	• Active urinary sediment with RBCs, WBCs, casts • Proteinuria, minimal, moderate, or heavy • Hypertension is common • May have azotemia or oliguria • May have edema
Histology	
Nonproliferative (GBM or podocyte disease, sclerosing)	• Proliferative histology - mesangial, epithelial, or endothelial cell proliferation, focal or diffuse • Glomerular inflammation mediated by infiltrating inflammatory cells • May have crescents in Bowman's space with parietal epithelial cell proliferation and fibrosis • May have glomerular vasculitis or thrombotic microangiopathy • May have mesangial, subendothelial, subepithelial or intramembranous immune deposits or anti-GBM antibody deposition

Nephrotic (cont.)	Nephritic
Differential diagnosis	
• Membranous nephropathy • Minimal change disease • Focal segmental glomerular sclerosis (FSGS) • Membranoproliferative GN (eg, hepatitis C, SLE) • Diabetic nephropathy • Amyloidosis **Less commonly:** • IgA nephropathy • Light chain deposition disease • Fibrillary GN • Hereditary nephritis (Alport syndrome)	• Poststreptococcal (postinfectious) GN • IgA nephropathy, Henoch-Schönlein purpura • Membranoproliferative GN (eg, hepatitis C, SLE) • Crescentic "rapidly progressive" GN (eg, ANCA-positive pauci-immune GN, granulomatosis with polyangiitis (formerly Wegener's granulomatosis), anti-GBM antibody GN or Goodpasture's syndrome) • HUS/TTP • Vasculitis (eg, polyarteritis nodosa, cryoglobulinemia) • Hereditary nephritis (Alport syndrome)

Initial tests
In patient with suspected glomerulonephritis (nephrotic or nephritic syndromes) • Complement levels (C3, C4) • ANA • ANCA (if rapidly progressive GN or vasculitis is suspected) • Anti-GBM antibody (if rapidly progressive GN) • Urine and plasma protein electrophoresis to assess source of proteinuria: UPEP (if >70% is albumin-glomerular proteinuria; if mainly globulins with multiple "polyclonal" peaks-tubular proteinuria; if single "monoclonal" globulin peak - prerenal "overflow" proteinuria due to monoclonal gammopathy) • Renal ultrasound to evaluate kidney size (small kidneys = chronicity), r/o PKD, obstructive or reflux nephropathy) **More specific tests:** • Antistreptococcal antibodies • Hepatitis B and C serology • HIV antibody • Cryoglobulins (must deliver warm blood to laboratory to avoid false-negative result) • VDRL

Serum complement components C3 and C4

C3 and C4 are useful initial tests to narrow the differential diagnosis of glomerular disease.

Decreased serum complement
• Poststreptococcal GN (complement returns to normal in 2-3 months)
• Peri-infectious GN: Subacute bacterial endocarditis, infected ventriculo-atrial "shunt" nephritis
• Membranoproliferative GN (complement stays low)
• SLE
• Cryoglobulinemia (complement often low)
• May be seen at times in HUS/TTP, rheumatoid vasculitis, atheroembolic disease

Normal serum complement
• Minimal change disease
• FSGS
• Membranous nephropathy
• IgA nephropathy, Henoch-Schönlein purpura
• Antiglomerular basement membrane disease
• Pauci-immune RPGN (ANCA positive or negative)
• Vasculitis: Granulomatosis with polyangiitis (Wegener's), polyarteritis nodosa
• Hereditary nephritis (Alport syndrome)

7.1 Nephrotic Syndrome

Minimal Change	Focal Segmental Glomerular Sclerosis	Membranous Glomerulopathy
Potential causes		

• **Idiopathic** most common
• **Secondary causes:**
  – Drugs, eg, NSAIDs, lithium, pamidronate
  – Hodgkin's disease, non-Hodgkin's lymphoma, leukemias
  – Acute variant of IgA nephropathy
	• **Idiopathic** most common (particularly in African Americans who may have an APOL1 allelic genetic risk)
	• **Secondary causes:**
	  – HIV nephropathy
	  – Heroin nephropathy
	  – Ureteral reflux nephropathy
	  – Sickle cell disease
	  – Malignancy (lymphomas)
	  – Transplant rejection
	  – Drugs: Lithium, anabolic steroids, pamidronate, interferon, adriamycin
	  – Secondary to other glomerulopathies (often without the nephrotic syndrome)
	  – Reduced renal mass and glomerulomegaly: Hyperfiltration due to underlying renal injury or obesity
		• **Idiopathic** most common. It appears that the majority of idiopathic cases have autoantibodies, mainly IgG4, directed against the phospholipase A2 receptor (PLA2R) in glomerular podocytes
		• **Secondary causes:**
		  – SLE
		  – Hepatitis B or C
		  – Malignancy (solid tumors, lymphomas)
		  – Sarcoidosis, rheumatoid arthritis, Sjögren syndrome
		  – Syphilis, malaria
		  – Drugs: Penicillamine, gold, NSAIDs, clopidogrel
		  – Sickle cell disease
		  – HIV

Pathology		
• **LM*:** Normal glomeruli, no interstitial disease • **IF:** No immune deposition • **EM:** Diffuse effacement or fusion of visceral epithelial foot processes	• **LM*:** Focal segmental glomerular sclerosis, mesangial hypercellularity, endocapillary foam cells, tubulo-interstitial disease • **IF:** Either no immune deposition or segmental deposits of IgM and C3 in the area of scarring • **EM:** Effacement or fusion of visceral epithelial foot processes, usually less diffuse in secondary FSGS	• **LM*:** Thickened glomerular basement membranes (GBMs) diffusely • **IF:** IgG & C3 in fine granular distribution along all GBMs • **EM:** Subepithelial electron-dense deposits in all GBMs

*LM: Light microscopy; **IF:** Immunofluorescent microscopy; **EM:** Electron microscopy.

General Principles of Nephrotic Syndrome Treatment		
Treatment of underlying disease	**Treatment of complications**	**Treatment of proteinuria**
• Specific to the type of glomerular disease (see below)	• Edema: Sodium restriction, • diuretics • Hyperlipidemia: Statins, fibrates • Hypercoagulability: Heparin followed by warfarin in those with a documented thrombotic or embolic event as long as heavy proteinuria persists	• ACEI or ARB, aliskiren if intolerant • Blood pressure control • Spironolactone (unproven)

7.2 Nephritic Syndrome

Mesangial Proliferative or Focal Proliferative GN	Poststreptococcal GN
IgA nephropathy, Henoch-Schönlein purpura, IgM nephropathy (variant of minimal change disease) • IgA nephropathy or Henoch-Schönlein purpura may present concomitantly with upper respiratory tract or other infections	• >10 days after infection with group A β-hemolytic Streptococcus
Pathology	
• **LM:** Mesangial cell proliferation • **IF:** Glomerular IgA deposits, frequently with C3 and sometimes IgG or IgM deposits • **EM:** Electron-dense deposits in the glomerular mesangium	• **LM:** Enlarged hypercellular glomeruli, endothelial cell proliferation, polymorphs in glomeruli • **IF:** Deposits of IgG, C3, sometimes IgM, IgA in glomerular capillaries & mesangium • **EM:** Scattered, large electro-dense subepithelial deposits "humps" & subendothelial deposits in glomerular capillaries

Membranoproliferative or Mesangio-capillary GN	Crescentic (rapidly progressive) GN
• **Immune complex deposition (usually type 1 or 3):** - Hepatitis C (with or without cryoglobulins) - SLE - Infections (endocarditis, abscess, parasitic diseases) - Monoclonal gammopathy (CLL, lymphomas) • **Complement deposition (usually type 2):** - Dense deposit disease - Disordered complement conditions • **No immune complex or complement deposition:** - Transplant nephropathy - Antiphospholipid syndrome - HUS/TTP	• **Type 1** - Anti-GBM antibodies (Goodpasture's syndrome) - 20% • **Type 2** - Immune complex deposition (SLE, crescentic IgA nephropathy, postinfectious GN, membranous, membranoproliferative GN, Henoch-Schönlein purpura) - 30-40% • **Type 3** - No immune deposition - pauci-immune (granulomatosis with polyangiitis (Wegener's), microscopic polyarteritis, polyarteritis nodosa) - 40-50%
Pathology	
• MPGN has several histologies defined by either immune deposition or electron microscopy findings - see chart of MPGN Pathology in section below.	• **LM:** Extensive crescent formation (extracapillary proliferation in Bowman's space of the glomeruli) • **IF:** - **Type 1** - linear GBM localization of Ig - **Type 2** - granular localization of glomerular immune complexes and complement - **Type 3** - no or scanty glomerular immunoglobulin deposition

7.3 IgA Nephropathy

IgA nephropathy, a common glomerulonephritis formerly considered to be a benign disease, is now recognized as a chronic kidney disease with as many as 40% progressing to ESRD. Predictors of a poor prognosis, dialysis or death, are as follows: Hypertension or impaired renal function at presentation, proteinuria ≥1 g/24h or nephrotic syndrome, older age, or severe pathologic lesions, such as crescents, on biopsy. Blood pressure control and reduction of proteinuria reduce the risk of death or dialysis.

7.3.1 Conditions associated with glomerular IgA deposits

- **Idiopathic IgA nephropathy is most common**
- **Henoch–Schönlein purpura**
- **Gastrointestinal**
  - Hepatic cirrhosis
  - Celiac disease
  - Inflammatory bowel disease
- **Rheumatologic**
  - Behcet's syndrome
  - Rheumatoid arthritis
  - Ankylosing spondylitis
  - Psoriatic arthritis
  - Reiter's syndrome
  - Relapsing polychondritis
- **Neoplastic**
  - Renal cell carcinoma
  - Non-Hodgkin's lymphoma
  - Bronchogenic carcinoma
  - Mesothelioma

- **Infectious**
  - Epstein-Barr virus
  - HIV
  - Osteomyelitis
  - Mycoplasma pneumoniae
  - Tuberculosis, leprosy, brucella
- **Dermatologic**
  - Psoriasis
  - Erythema nodosum
  - Dermatitis herpetiformis
- **Ophthalmologic**
  - Uveitis
  - Scleritis
- **Miscellaneous**
  - Granulomatosis with polyangiitis (Wegener's)
  - Familial Mediterranean fever
  - Myasthenia
  - Hemochromatosis
  - Sarcoidosis

7.3.2   Treatment of IgA

Treatment of IgA Nephropathy or Henoch-Schönlein Purpura		
Proteinuria <1g/ 24h	Proteinura 1–3g/ 24h	Proteinuria >3g/24h
• No treatment - observation • ACEI or ARB for hypertension	• Observation with normal renal function • ACEI or ARB • Fish oil 12 g/day with renal insufficiency may be somewhat helpful	• ACEI or ARB • If progressing disease & eGFR >50 ml/min, corticosteroids, eg, prednisone 1 mg/Kg/day on alternative days for 8 wks then taper in responders • Immunosuppressives (cyclophosphamide, azathioprine) & other Rx (see below) • If eGFR < 50 ml/min or no response, fish oil 12 g/day may be tried to slow progression
Other therapeutic options for IgA nephropathy or HSP		
• Crescentic IgA nephropathy: pulse corticosteroids/plasmapheresis/immunosuppressives • High dose IV immune globulin in severe IgA or Henoch-Schönlein purpura • Antiplatelet medications (dipyridamole), heparin, warfarin • Tonsillectomy with or without pulse corticosteroids		

7.4   Membranous Nephropathy

Membranous nephropathy is the most common form of nephrotic syndrome in adults. In 1/4 of cases it is caused by an underlying disease (see chart of Nephrotic Syndrome above for causes). Approximately 1/3 of patients have a spontaneous remission, 1/3 remain stable, and 1/3 progress to ESRD.

Histologic features that help to differentiate primary (idiopathic) from secondary membranous nephropathy
• Positive staining for IgG4 in primary nephropathy, while IgG1 and IgG3 may be found in SLE or IgG1 and IgG2 with malignancies
• Increased staining for the PLA2 receptor in glomeruli correlates with antibodies to PLA2 receptor, consistent with primary membranous nephropathy
• Subepithelial and intramembranous deposits characterize primary nephropathy, while mesangial or subendothelial deposits or tubular immune staining may be found in secondary nephropathy

Membranous Nephropathy: Treatment

Treatment of Membranous Nephropathy

Decision to treat is based upon adverse risk profile

Risk factors for progression to renal failure:
- Severe nephrotic syndrome
- Hypertension
- Age over 50 years
- Male sex
- Renal insufficiency at presentation

Symptomatic treatment of nephrotic syndrome as noted above for stable and low-risk disease

Cytotoxic therapy (x3 cycles) for primary membranous nephropathy

- Methylprednisolone 1g IV x 3 days
- Prednisone 0.4 mg/Kg/day PO x 27 days
- Then chlorambucil 0.2 mg/Kg/day PO x 28 days (or cyclophosphamide 2.5 mg/Kg/day in months 2, 4, and 6 is usually better tolerated than chlorambucil)

Review at 6–12 months

- If positive response – taper treatment
- No response – change to cyclosporine therapy 3.5 mg/Kg/day x 12 months or one of newer options below

Other therapeutic options for membranous nephropathy:

- Cyclosporine (4–5 mg/Kg/day) in 6-month cycles, each followed by a one-month washout. Initiate subsequent cycle if proteinuria rises into nephrotic range during washout period.
- Add cytotoxic agent (e.g. mycophenolate mofetil) from the third cyclosporine cycle onwards in those with persistent relapses
- Mycophenolate mofetil
- Rituximab is a newer potential alternative & may become a first-line therapy
- ACTH
- IV immune globulin

7.5   Focal Segmental Glomerular Sclerosis (FSGS)

FSGS may present as a primary (idiopathic) disease or secondary to an underlying disorder with treatment dependent on managing the primary cause.

Negative prognostic indicators
- ↑ Creatinine at diagnosis (>1.3 mg/dL)
- Nephrotic range proteinuria
- Hypertension
- Interstitial fibrosis (≥20%) on biopsy

Features Differentiating Primary from Secondary FSGS	
Primary (idiopathic)	**Secondary**
Presentation • Characterized by sudden onset, presence of edema & hypoalbuminemia, **Histologic forms** • Cellular, collapsing glomerulopathy, or glomerular tip lesion • Podocytes are uniformly effaced **Treatment** • See below	**Causes** • See chart of Nephrotic Syndrome above for causes **Presentation** • Slow onset • Absence of edema and hypoalbuminemia **Histology** • Enlarged glomeruli • Heterogenous effacement of podocytes **Treatment** • ACEI or ARB • Blood pressure control • Treatment of underlying cause, eg, HAART Rx for HIV, weight loss for morbid obesity

Treatment of Primary FSGS
Corticosteroid therapy
• Prednisone 0.5-2 mg/Kg/day (remission associated with ≥60 mg/d for 3 months). If positive response ⇒ ↓ to 0.5 mg/Kg/day and treat for another 1.5-2 months, then taper over 1-1.5 months. In the elderly (>60y) 1.0-1.6 mg/Kg (up to 100 mg) every other day for 3-5 months • Treat for 6 months before defining as steroid-resistant

Treatment of Primary FSGS (cont.)

Mild or moderate disease - (proteinuria 0.5-2.0 g/24 h proteinuria, stable creatinine):

- ACEI or ARB
- Blood pressure control
- Sodium restriction & diuretics, if needed
- CVD risk factor management, eg, statins

Steroid-resistant cases

- Cyclosporine 5-10 mg/Kg/day (to maintain whole blood trough level of 100-200 ng/ml) for 6 months, then reduce by 25% every 2 months for a total of 12 months. Relapses after stopping or reducing the dose are common
- Cytotoxic therapy (cyclophosphamide, azathioprine, chlorambucil) - inconclusive evidence

Relapse

- If relapse after prolonged remission - repeat a course of steroids
- Frequent relapsers/steroid dependent - steroids (1 mg/kg/d up to 80 mg/d for up to 1 month, then taper over 1 month) + cyclosporine (5-6 mg/kg/day) or cytotoxics (limited to 3 month course)

Other therapeutic options for FSGS

- Calcineurin inhibitors (cyclosporine, tacrolimus) or cytotoxic therapy as above instead of steroids
- Mycophenolate mofetil
- Sirolimus
- Plasmapheresis or protein adsorption for kidney transplant patients with recurrent FSGS

7.6 Minimal Change Disease (MCD)

Minimal change disease is the most common cause of nephrotic syndrome in children, but less common in adults (10-15% of nephrotic syndrome). Similar to other nephrotic diseases, MCD can be idiopathic (primary) which is by far the more common or secondary to underlying disorders (eg, associated with neoplastic diseases, toxic or allergic reactions to drugs, infections, auto-immune disorders). However, primary and secondary MCD presents similarly, and the histologic features of effacement of foot processes on electron microscopy, but no changes on light microscopy, are similar. In some cases, particularly in older patients, MCD can present with acute renal failure accompanying the nephrotic syndrome, with reversibility upon successful treatment.

Treatment of Minimal Change Disease

Corticosteroid therapy

- Prednisone 60 mg/m^2/day (up to 80 mg/day) for 4-6 weeks (or 120 mg/m^2 up to 150 mg every other day)
- If positive response, taper dose - 40 mg/m^2/day every alternate day for 4-6 weeks until urine is protein free then taper off

Mild disease: Nonspecific treatment of nephrotic syndrome

- ACEI or ARB
- Blood pressure control
- Sodium restriction & diuretics, if needed
- CVD risk factor management, eg, statins

Relapse

Prednisone 60 mg/m^2/day (up to 80 mg/day) until urine protein free, then 40 mg/m^2 on alternate days for 4 wks

Steroid-resistant cases

- If steroid resistant: No response to initial treatment (60 mg/m^2/day for 4-6 wks)
- Or if frequent relapses
- Or if steroid dependent
- Consider other therapeutic options below

Other therapeutic options for MCD

- Cyclophosphamide 2 mg/Kg/day for 8 weeks
- In steroid resistant or dependent - cyclosporine 5 mg/Kg/day (in children 6 mg/Kg/day) for 6-12 months
- In cases with frequent relapses:
  - Chlorambucil 0.15 mg/kg/day with tapering alternate day prednisone for 8 wks
  - Levamisole
  - Long-term alternate day prednisone
- Alternative/newer therapies:
  - Mycophenolate mofetil
  - Rituximab

7.7 Membranoproliferative GN (MPGN)

Patients with MPGN may have a nephritic and/or nephrotic presentation

7.7.1 MPGN: Pathology

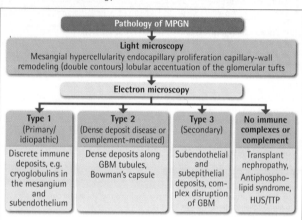

Pathology of MPGN

Light microscopy
Mesangial hypercellularity endocapillary proliferation capillary-wall remodeling (double contours) lobular accentuation of the glomerular tufts

Electron microscopy

Type 1 (Primary/ idiopathic)	**Type 2** (Dense deposit disease or complement-mediated)	**Type 3** (Secondary)	**No immune complexes or complement**
Discrete immune deposits, e.g. cryoglobulins in the mesangium and subendothelium	Dense deposits along GBM tubules, Bowman's capsule	Subendothelial and subepithelial deposits, complex disruption of GBM	Transplant nephropathy, Antiphospholipid syndrome, HUS/TTP

7.7.2   MPGN: Pathophysiology

Pathophysiology
MPGN type 1 and MPGN type 3 may be immune-complex–mediated and/or complement-mediated; MPGN type 2 appears to be C3 mediated, e.g., by C3 nephritic factor

Immune complex mediated (increased levels of circulating immune complexes triggers activation of classical complement pathway)	**Complement mediated** (dysregulation of alternative complement pathway activation with C3 deposition)
• Chronic infections (viral, bacterial, fungal, parasitic), Hepatitis B or C • Autoimmune diseases (SLE, Sjögren's syndrome, rheumatoid arthritis, and mixed connective-tissue disorders) • Paraproteinemias due to monoclonal gammopathies (multiple myeloma, lymphomas, CLL, MGUS)	• Underlying factors H and B genetic polymorphisms. • Membrane cofactor protein, and C3 genetic poly-morphisms

7.8 Poststreptococcal or Postinfectious GN

PSGN or PIGN: Most cases of PSGN have a relatively benign disease, or are at least reversible. The symptoms should resolve in a few weeks, and C3 should normalize in 6-8 weeks (kidney biopsy becomes indicated for persistent disease to rule out MPGN or SLE). However, some patients develop crescentic disease with a rapid decline in renal function, and rarely, patients develop CKD with persistent hematuria, proteinuria, and decline in renal function.

Diagnostic tests

Since the most common pathogen causing PIGN is group A beta-hemolytic Streptococcus infection occurring > 10 days previously, tests indicating the exposure are helpful in diagnosis
- Anti-DNase B (antibodies to a product of group A Strep)
- Serum ASO (antibodies against streptolysin O)

Non-specific tests to help diagnostically
- Serum complement levels - expect low C3 and C4
- Kidney biopsy - pathology as noted in Nephritic Syndrome chart

Treatment of PIGN	
Non-specific Therapy	**Immunosuppressive Therapy**
• Blood pressure control • Treat fluid overload and edema - sodium restriction, diuretics • Supportive treatment with temporary dialysis, if needed • Treat infection (if still present)	• Corticosteroids for crescentic disease

7.9 Crescentic GN

Crescent formation indicates severe injury of the glomerular capillary wall with fibrin leak into Bowman's space, parietal epithelial cell proliferation, and phagocyte migration, leading to crescent formation.

Clinically crescentic GN usually presents with rapid progression of acute or subacute renal failure (rapidly progressive GN). Many forms of glomerular disease may present with crescent formation, necrotizing glomerular lesions, and rapid progression (see below).

Crescentic GN		
Type 1	Type 2	Type 3
Caused by antibodies against the GBM: Anti-GBM nephritis or Goodpasture's syndrome (linear deposition along the GBM)	Caused by glomerular deposition of immune complexes, frequently RPGN superimposed on a primary glomerular disease: Crescentic IgA nephropathy, HSP, membranoproliferative GN, hepatitis B or C nephropathy, cryoglobulinemia, SLE, poststreptococcal or post-infectious GN, amyloidosis, multiple myeloma	Pauci-immune - no or scant immune deposition: ANCA-associated vasculitides, granulomatosis with polyangiitis (Wegener's), microscopic polyarteritis, Churg-Strauss syndrome, medication associated (propylthiouracil, allopurinol, penicillamine, hydralazine, others), ANCA-negative RPGN, polyarteritis nodosa

Treatment of Crescentic GN

Anti-GBM Ab - linear staining on IF

SCr <6 mg/dL (< ~600 mcmol/L), <85% crescents on biopsy

- Therapeutic plasma exchange (TPE) - daily 4 L plasma exchange for 7 days then daily or alternate day for 7-14 days or until anti-GBM Ab titer low or negative
- Pulse methylprednisolone + prednisone - 7-15 mg/Kg/day (maximum 1 g/day) for 3 days, then prednisone 60 mg/day tapered weekly
- Cyclophosphamide - for <55 years old: 3 mg/kg/day (down to nearest 50 mg) for 8 wks; for >55 years old: 2 mg/kg/day for 8 weeks
- Prolonged Rx if anti-GBM Ab remains detectable

Anti-GBM Ab - linear staining on IF

SCr > 6 mg/dL (>~600 mcmol/L), >85% crescents on biopsy

- Prognosis for renal recovery is poor so risk: benefit assessment of aggressive Rx is warranted
- Supportive therapy with dialysis may be best
- For pulmonary hemorrhage - TPE ± immune suppressive Rx

Immune complex deposition - granular localization

Treatment based on specific glomerular disorder

Pauci-immune

- Pulse methylprednisolone + prednisone - 7-15 mg/Kg/day (maximum 1 g/day) for 3 days, then prednisone 1 mg/kg/day for 1 month, gradually tapered over 6-12 months
- Cyclophosphamide - Oral dose of 2 mg/Kg/day for 8 wks, adjust to WBC ≥3,000-5,000. Alternatively, IV dose: 0.5 g/m^2/month and increase monthly to 0.75 g/m^2/month then a maximum of 1.0 g/m^2/month, if needed - control WBC count ≥3,000-5,000 two weeks after dose
- TPE can be added with pulmonary hemorrhage or if no response to above Rx

References and Suggested Reading

Nephrotic/Nephritic Syndromes

Kodner C. Nephrotic syndrome in adults: diagnosis and management. Am Fam Physician 2009;80:1129-34.

Zhang S, Audard V, Fan Q, Pawlak A, Lang P, Sahali D. Immunopathogenesis of idiopathic nephrotic syndrome. Contrib Nephrol 2011;169:94-106.

McGrogan A, Franssen CF, de Vries CS. The incidence of primary glomerulonephritis worldwide: a systematic review of the literature. Nephrol Dial Transplant 2011;26:414-30.

Kashtan CE. Alport syndrome. An inherited disorder of renal, ocular, and cochlear basement membranes. Medicine (Baltimore) 1999; 78(5):338-60.

IgA Nephropathy

Boyd JK, Cheung CK, Molyneux K, et al. An update on the pathogenesis and treatment of IgA nephropathy. Kidney Int 2012; 81(9):833-43.

Lv J, Xu D, Perkovic V, et al; HYPERLINK "http://www.ncbi.nlm.nih.gov/pubmed?term=TEST-ING%20Study%20Group%5BCorporate%20Author%5D" TESTING Study Group. Corticosteroid therapy in IgA nephropathy. Am Soc J Nephrol 2012; 23(6):1108-16.

Kamei K, Nakanishi K, Ito S, et al. Long-term results of a randomized controlled trial in childhood IgA nephropathy. Clin J Am Soc Nephrol 2011;6:1301-7.

Nakagawa N, Kabara M, Matsuki M, et al. Retrospective Comparison of the Efficacy of Tonsillectomy with and without Steroid-pulse Therapy in IgA Nephropathy Patients. Intern Med 2012;51:1323-8.

Imai H, Miura N. A treatment dilemma in adult immunoglobulin A nephropathy: what is the appropriate target, preservation of kidney function or induction of clinical remission? Clin Exp Nephrol 2011;16: 195-201.

Berthoux F, Mohey H, Laurent B, Mariat C, Afiani A, Thibaudin L. Predicting the risk for dialysis or death in IgA nephropathy. J Am Soc Nephrol 2011;22:752-61.

Zhou YH, Tang LG, Guo SL, et al. Steroids in the treatment of IgA nephropathy to the improvement of renal survival: a systematic review and meta-analysis. PLoS One 2011;6:e18788.

Fawole A, Daw H, Taylor H, Rashidi A. Immunoglobulin A nephropathy associated with mesothelioma. WMJ 2012;111:29-32.

Floege J, Eitner F. Current therapy for IgA nephropathy. J Am Soc Nephrol 2011;22:1785-94.

Membranous Nephropathy

Ponticelli C, Passerini P. Can prognostic factors assist therapeutic decisions in idiopathic membranous nephropathy? J Nephrol 2010;23:156-63.

Bomback AS, Derebail VK, McGregor JG, Kshirsagar AV, Falk RJ, Nachman PH. Rituximab therapy for membranous nephropathy: a systematic review. Clin J Am Soc Nephrol 2009;4:734-44.

Cattran D. Management of membranous nephropathy: when and what for treatment. J Am Soc Nephrol 2005;16:1188-94.

Ponticelli C. Membranous nephropathy. J Nephrol 2007;20:268-87.

Beck LH Jr, Bonegio RG, Lambeau G, et al. M-type phospholipase A2 receptor as target antigen in idiopathic membranous nephropathy. N Engl J Med 2009; 361(1):11-21.

Appel GB. Rituximab in membranous nephropathy: Is it a first-line treatment? J Am Soc Nephrol 2012; 23(8): 1280-2.

Hoxha E, Kneibler U, Stege g, et al. Enhanced expression of the M-type phospholipase A2 receptor in glomeruli correlates with serum receptor antibodies in primary membranous nephropathy. Kidney Int 2012; 82(7):797-804.

References and Suggested Reading (cont.)

Focal Segmental Glomerular Sclerosis

Cameron JS. Focal segmental glomerulosclerosis in adults. Nephrol Dial Transplant 2003;18 Suppl 6: vi45-51.

Genovese G, Friedman DJ, Ross MD, et al. Association of trypanolytic ApoL1 variants with kidney disease in African Americans. Science 2010;329:841-5.

Genovese G, Tonna SJ, Knob AU, et al. A risk allele for focal segmental glomerulosclerosis in African Americans is located within a region containing APOL1 and MYH9. Kidney Int 2010;78:698-704.

Minimal Change Disease

Waldman M, Crew RJ, Valeri A, et al. Adult minimal-change disease: clinical characteristics, treatment, and outcomes. Clin J Am Soc Nephrol 2007; 2(3): 445-53.

Glassock RJ. Secondary minimal change disease. Nephrol Dial Transplant 2003;18 Suppl 6:vi52-8.

Membranoproliferative Glomerulopathy

Sethi S, Fervenza FC. Membranoproliferative glomerulonephritis--a new look at an old entity. N Engl J Med 2012;366:1119-31.

Sethi S, Nester CM, Smith RJ. Membranoproliferative glomerulonephritis and C3 glomerulopathy: resolving the confusion. Kidney Int 2011;81:434-41.

Sethi S, Fervenza FC. Membranoproliferative glomerulonephritis: pathogenetic heterogeneity and proposal for a new classification. Semin Nephrol 2011;31:341-8.

Poststreptoccal/Postinfectious Glomerulonephritis

Nast CC. Infection-related glomerulonephritis: changing demographics and outcomes. Adv Chronic Kidney Dis 2012;19:68-75.

Nadasdy T, Hebert LA. Infection-related glomerulonephritis: understanding mechanisms. Semin Nephrol 2011;31:369-75.

Brodsky SV, Nadasdy T. Infection-related glomerulonephritis. Contrib Nephrol 2011; 169:153-60.

Crescentic Glomerulopathy (Rapidly Progressive Glomerulonephritis)

Jennette JC. Rapidly progressive crescentic glomerulonephritis. Kidney Int 2003; 63(3):1164-77.

Seo P, Stone JH. The antineutrophil cytoplasmic antibody-associated vasculitides. Am J Med 2004; 117(1):39-50.

Chen M, Yu F, Wang SX, et al. Antineutrophil cytoplasmic autoantibody-negative pauci-immune crescentic glomerulonephritis. J Am Soc Nephrol 2007; 18(2):599-605.

Lionaki S, Jennette JC, Falk RJ. Anti-neutrophil cytoplasmic (ANCA) and anti-glomerular basement membrane (GBM) autoantibodies in necrotizing and crescentic glomerulonephritis. Semin Immunopathol 2007; 29(4):459-74.

Crosthwaite A, Skene A, Mount P. Rapidly progressive glomerulonephritis complicating primary AL amyloidosis and multiple myeloma. Nephrol Dial Transplant 2010;25:2786-9.

Bajema IM. Pathological classification of anti-neutrophil cytoplasmic antibody (ANCA)-associated glomerulonephritis. Clin Exp Immunol 2011;164 Suppl 1:14-6.

Tarzi RM, Cook HT, Pusey CD. Crescentic glomerulonephritis: new aspects of pathogenesis. Semin Nephrol 2011;31:361-8.

8 Various Kidney Diseases: Interstitial, Cystic, Obstructive, & Infectious Diseases

8.1 Acute Interstitial Nephritis (AIN)

AIN histopathology includes edema and infiltration of the renal interstitium with inflammatory cells (mononuclear cells, T-lymphocytes, plasma cells, and eosinophils), while the glomeruli and blood vessels are usually spared. AIN can eventually lead to interstitial fibrosis (chronic interstitial nephritis).

8.1.1 Causes of AIN

- **'Allergic' interstitial nephritis** (most commonly drug-induced)
  - Proton pump inhibitors
  - NSAIDs (may be accompanied by MCD nephrotic syndrome)
  - Antibiotics (eg, beta-lactams, rifampin, sulfa, ciprofloxacin)
  - Allopurinol
  - Mesalamine
  - Cimetidine
- **Toxins**
  - Many of the drugs and chemicals listed below as causes of chronic interstitial nephritis can cause AIN as well

- **Infections**
  - Acute bacterial pyelonephritis (polymorphonuclear leukocytes predominate)
  - Leptospirosis
  - Legionella
  - Tuberculosis
  - Streptococcus, beta-hemolytic (Councilman's nephritis)
  - Viral - cytomegalovirus, EBV, BK (polyoma) virus, HIV
- **Autoimmune disorders**
  - SLE
  - Sarcoidosis
  - Sjögren's syndrome
  - Tubulointerstitial nephritis-uveitis (TINU) syndrome

8.1.2   Clinical presentation of allergic interstitial nephritis

- **'Full-blown' presentation:** Fever, rash, arthralgias, and renal insufficiency but typically not all features are present
- **UA:** Subnephrotic proteinuria, mild hematuria, WBCs, often with eosinophiluria
- **Blood count:** Eosinophilia and anemia may be present
- **Blood chemistries:** ARF, may have acidosis and hyperkalemia and, at times, elevated liver enzymes

8.1.3   Diagnosis of allergic interstitial nephritis

- Kidney biopsy is the gold standard
- Gallium-67 renal scan uptake in AIN may distinguish it from ATN when biopsy is undesirable or contraindicated
- Response to discontinuation of the suspected offending agent and a therapeutic trial of corticosteroids over 1-2 weeks may be used to make a presumptive diagnosis

8.1.4   Treatment of AIN

- Treatment aimed at identifying and discontinuing specific offending agents above, if possible
- Discontinue all possible offending medications that aren't essential, if no known cause identified
- Supportive care of ARF (manage volume status and electrolytes)
- Role of steroids is unproven, but if used, 40-60 mg (or 1 mg/Kg) per day of oral prednisone for 2-3 weeks, then taper over 3-4 weeks

8.2 Chronic Interstitial Nephritis

Chronic interstitial nephritis is a large and heterogeneous category of diseases leading primarily to interstitial fibrosis and tubular atrophy. Since progressive, sclerosing kidney diseases of all types are associated with eventual interstitial fibrosis and tubular atrophy, it is useful to define chronic interstitial nephritis as those conditions that cause interstitial and tubular damage initially while leaving glomeruli and vasculature intact.

8.2.1 Causes of chronic interstitial nephritis

- Infection
  - Pyelonephritis
  - HIV
  - TB
  - EBV
  - BK (polyoma) virus
- Anatomic diseases
  - Obstructive uropathy
  - Nephronophthisis
  - Congenital disorders
- Drug/chemical-induced
  - Lithium nephropathy
  - Analgesic nephropathy (>2-3 Kg total intake)
  - Calcineurin inhibitors
  - Chemotherapy (cisplatin, ifosfamide, nitrosoureas)
  - Cocaine and heroin
  - Lead, cadmium, mercury
  - Balkan nephropathy
  - Chinese herbal (aristolochic acid) nephropathy

- Immunologic diseases
  - SLE
  - Sarcoidosis
  - Sjögren's syndrome
  - Rheumatoid arthritis
  - IgG4-associated AIN
  - Tubulointerstitial nephritis and uveitis (TINU syndrome)
- Metabolic disorders
  - Nephrocalcinosis
  - Oxalosis
  - Gouty nephropathy
  - Hypokalemic nephropathy
- Other
  - Consequence of unresolved AIN or ATN
  - Radiation nephritis
  - Myeloma kidney, lymphoma
  - Sickle cell disease
  - Mitochondrial cytopathies

8.3 Interstitial Fibrosis

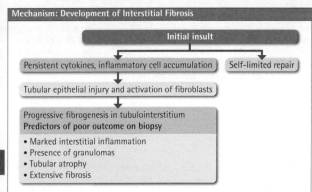

Mechanism: Development of Interstitial Fibrosis

Initial insult

Persistent cytokines, inflammatory cell accumulation   Self-limited repair

Tubular epithelial injury and activation of fibroblasts

Progressive fibrogenesis in tubulointerstitium
Predictors of poor outcome on biopsy

• Marked interstitial inflammation
• Presence of granulomas
• Tubular atrophy
• Extensive fibrosis

8.4   Role of NSAIDs in Kidney Disease

Non-steroidal anti-inflammatory drugs (NSAIDs) are probably one of the most commonly used medications as they are available over the counter. NSAIDs can affect the kidneys in several ways.

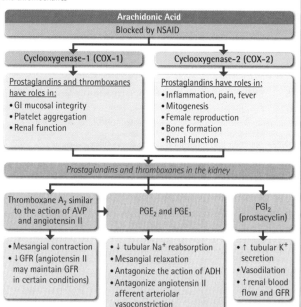

Mechanism: Action of NSAID's

Inhibit cyclooxygenase enzymatic conversion of arachidonate to prostaglandins and thromboxanes

Arachidonic Acid
Blocked by NSAID

Cyclooxygenase-1 (COX-1)

Prostaglandins and thromboxanes have roles in:
• GI mucosal integrity
• Platelet aggregation
• Renal function

Cyclooxygenase-2 (COX-2)

Prostaglandins have roles in:
• Inflammation, pain, fever
• Mitogenesis
• Female reproduction
• Bone formation
• Renal function

Prostaglandins and thromboxanes in the kidney

Thromboxane A_2 similar to the action of AVP and angiotensin II

• Mesangial contraction
• ↓GFR (angiotensin II may maintain GFR in certain conditions)

PGE_2 and PGE_1

• ↓ tubular Na^+ reabsorption
• Mesangial relaxation
• Antagonize the action of ADH
• Antagonize angiotensin II afferent arteriolar vasoconstriction

PGI_2 (prostacyclin)

• ↑ tubular K^+ secretion
• Vasodilation
• ↑ renal blood flow and GFR

Renal effects of NSAIDs	
Decreased PGE_2 can cause:	Decreased PGI_2 (prostacyclin) can cause:
• Sodium retention • Peripheral edema • ↑ BP • CHF (rarely)	• Hyperkalemia • ↓ Renal blood flow and GFR (may lead to ARF) • Hyperreninemic hypoaldosteronism

Renal Insufficiency Mechanisms Of NSAID's	
Acute	Chronic
• Acute interstitial nephritis • ATN • Hemodynamic compromise	• Nephrotic syndrome - minimal change disease • Chronic tubulointerstitial disease • Papillary necrosis

8.5   PKD & Other Hereditary Cystic Kidney Diseases

8.5.1   Hereditary cystic kidney diseases

- Autosomal dominant polycystic kidney disease (ADPKD)
- Autosomal recessive polycystic kidney disease
- Nephronophthisis (NPHP)-Medullary Cystic Kidney Disease complex
- Bardet-Biedl syndrome
- Oral-Facial-Digital syndrome
- Miscellaneous hereditary PKD syndromes
  - ADPKD associated with tuberous sclerosis
  - ADPKD associated with von Hippel-Lindau

8.5.2   Polycystic Kidney Disease (PKD)

PKD is relatively common (1 in every 400 to 1000 live births, accounts for 5–10% of ESRD). Most of patients with PKD also have liver cysts, but only a fraction of patients develop massive polycystic liver disease.

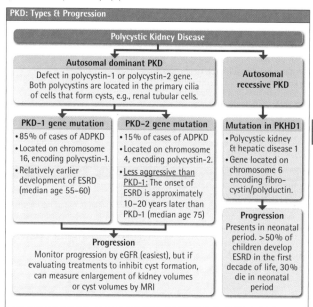

PKD: Types & Progression

Polycystic Kidney Disease

Autosomal dominant PKD
Defect in polycystin-1 or polycystin-2 gene. Both polycystins are located in the primary cilia of cells that form cysts, e.g., renal tubular cells.

Autosomal recessive PKD

PKD-1 gene mutation
- 85% of cases of ADPKD
- Located on chromosome 16, encoding polycystin-1.
- Relatively earlier development of ESRD (median age 55–60)

PKD-2 gene mutation
- 15% of cases of ADPKD
- Located on chromosome 4, encoding polycystin-2.
- Less aggressive than PKD-1: The onset of ESRD is approximately 10–20 years later than PKD-1 (median age 75)

Mutation in PKHD1
- Polycystic kidney & hepatic disease 1
- Gene located on chromosome 6 encoding fibrocystin/polyductin.

Progression
Presents in neonatal period. > 50% of children develop ESRD in the first decade of life, 30% die in neonatal period

Progression
Monitor progression by eGFR (easiest), but if evaluating treatments to inhibit cyst formation, can measure enlargement of kidney volumes or cyst volumes by MRI

8.5.3   Diagnosis of PKD

Diagnosis	
Family Hx, but no family Hx in 10-25% of cases	
Radiological (US, CT, MRI)	**Molecular**
Ultrasound criteria (based on age) in at risk (family Hx) patients: • 15-39 years: At least 3 unilateral or bilateral cysts • 40-59 years: 2 cysts in each kidney • >60 years: 4 cysts in each kidney • Fewer than 2 cysts in at-risk patients ≥40 years old usually excludes the disease. Without family Hx, >8-10 cysts in each kidney or concomitant liver cysts suggest PKD	• Genetic testing can identify only 70% of all PKD-1 and PKD-2 mutations • Linkage analysis to study family cases • Mutation analysis (exon sequencing)

8.5.4   Treatment of PKD

Treatments to Slow Progression of PKD	Potential Therapies
• Hypertension develops in most patients and is associated with progressive disease: ACEI or ARB drugs of choice for BP control	• V2 vasopressin receptor antagonist: Tolvaptan • The mammalian target of rapamycin (mTOR): mTOR inhibitors: sirolimus, everolimus • cAMP: Metformin (activates AMP-activated protein kinase) • Somatostatin

8.5.5 Medullary Cystic Disease

Characterized by family history, bilateral small cysts which when detected are often at the corticomedullary junction, tubulointerstitial sclerosis, kidneys of normal or small size, and progression to renal failure and ESRD. Gout or hyperuricemia and urinary concentrating defects are common whereas hypertension is not. It is inherited in an autosomal dominant pattern and can be diagnosed by genetic testing in families.

Type 1	Type 2
• Late onset (around 60 years old)	• Early onset (around 30 years old)
• Defect in MCKD1 gene	• Defect in MCKD2 gene (uromodulin/ Tamm-Horsfall mucoprotein)

Treatment
• No effective treatment exists
• Control of other renal risk factors and CKD symptoms
• Correction of water and electrolyte imbalances if present
• Therapy for gout/hyperuricemia if present

8.6 Obstructive Uropathy

8.6.1 Obstructive uropathy (obstruction to urine flow) can cause:

- Hydronephrosis (dilatation of the renal pelvis)
- Hydroureter(s)
- Bladder distention and dysfunction
- Nephropathy (renal damage from obstruction)
  - ARF: 5-10% of ARF is caused by high-grade obstruction
  - CKD: a small percentage is caused by long lasting obstruction
  - Hypertension
  - Distal renal tubular acidosis
  - Hyperkalemia

8.6.2 Causes of urinary tract obstruction

- Upper Urinary Tract Obstruction
  - Congenital ureteropelvic junction obstruction or horseshoe kidney
  - Kidney stones, blood clots, or sloughed renal papillae
  - Transitional cell carcinoma obstructing the renal pelvis or ureter
  - Retroperitoneal malignancy
  - Retroperitoneal fibrosis

- Lower Urinary Tract Obstruction
  - Benign prostatic hypertrophy or prostate cancer
  - Bladder cancer obstructing the bladder neck or ureter(s)
  - Bladder stones, blood clots, or fungal ball(s)
  - Neurogenic bladder
  - Urethral stricture or valves
  - Malpositioned Foley catheter
- Vesicoureteral reflux in children and young adults: Not a true obstructive uropathy, but high-grade reflux can cause hydronephrosis and reflux nephropathy, a secondary FSGS manifested by proteinuria and CKD

8.6.3 Diagnostic tests to evaluate or rule out obstruction

- Bladder catheterization
- Ultrasound (excellent screening study but sensitivity ranges from 80-95%, lower in early obstruction before renal pelvic dilatation has occurred)
- CT scan without or with radiocontrast
- Intravenous pyelography (IVP requires radiocontrast)
- Retrograde or antegrade pyelography
- Radioisotope renography

For evaluation of suspected vesicoureteral reflux, cystography can document and grade degree of retrograde reflux of radiocontrast from the bladder up the ureter(s).

8.6.4 Treatment

- For lower urinary tract obstruction: Bladder drainage (straight or Foley catheter or percutaneous suprapubic catheter placement)
- For upper urinary tract obstruction: Percutaneous nephrostomy or retrograde ureteral stent placement
- Eliminate the cause of obstruction, if possible (eg, remove kidney or bladder stones)
- Treat urinary tract infection if present.

8.7 Urinary Tract Infection (UTI)

Asymptomatic bacteriuria needs to be treated only in:
- Pregnant women
- Diabetics
- Neutropenic patients
- Transplant and other immune suppressed patients
- Before urologic procedures
- With obstruction, reflux, or other anatomic kidney conditions, eg, polycystic kidney disease

8.7.1   Types & Treatment of UTI

Type of UTI	Common Pathogens	Common Treatment Choices
Uncomplicated UTI/Cystitis		
• Symptoms: Dysuria, urinary urgency, frequency, lower abdominal pain • Findings: Hematuria or cloudy urine, positive leukocyte esterase & nitrites on dipstick, WBCs & bacteria in sediment microscopy	• E. Coli • Other Gram negatives • Staphylococcus saprophyticus • Enterococcus	• Nitrofurantoin 100 mg twice daily for 5 days • TMP/SMX double-strength twice a day for 3 days • Fluoroquinolone for 3 days • Beta-lactam for 3 days • In pregnancy: beta-lactam often used • In elderly, Rx for 3-7 days
Uncomplicated pyelonephritis		
Kidney infection without complicating factors noted for asymptomatic bacteriuria in 8.7 above • Symptoms: Fever, chills, flank pain, nausea/vomiting • Findings: CVA tenderness, >100,000 organisms /ml on culture	• E. Coli • Other Gram negatives • Staphylococcus saprophyticus • Enterococcus	• Fluoroquinolone for 7-10 days • Inpatient Rx: May substitute IV ampicillin & gentamicin or 3rd generation cephalosporin. • Treatment then guided by culture sensitivity for 7-10 days
Complicated pyelonephritis		
Kidney infection with a complicating factor noted for asymptomatic bacteriuria in 8.7 above	• E. Coli • Proteus mirabilis • Klebsiella pneumoniae • Pseudomonas aeruginosa • Staphylococcus aureus • Candida spp.	• Ampicillin+gentamicin IV • Fluoroquinolone IV initially • 3rd generation cephalosporin • Treatment then guided by culture sensitivity for 10-14 days • For yeast, fluconazole, amphotericin B, or if necessary, flucytosine

References and Suggested Reading

Acute interstitial nephritis

Kodner CM, Kudrimoti A. Diagnosis and management of acute interstitial nephritis. Am Fam Physician 2003;67:2527-34.

Rossert J. Drug-induced acute interstitial nephritis. Kidney Int 2001;60:804-17.

Schwarz A, Krause PH, Kunzendorf U, et al. The outcome of acute interstitial nephritis: risk factors for the transition from acute to chronic interstitial nephritis. Clin Nephrol 2000; 54(3):179-90.

Chronic interstitial nephritis

Zeisberg M, Neilson EG. Mechanisms of tubulointerstitial fibrosis. J Am Soc Nephrol 2010; 21:1819-34.

Eric G. Neilson Interstitial nephritis: another kissing disease? J Clin Invest. 1999; 104(12): 1671-1672.

Becker J, Miller F, Nuovo GJ, et al. Epstein-Barr virus infection of renal proximal tubule cells: possible role in chronic interstitial nephritis. J Clin Invest 1999; 104(12):1673-1681.

Stone JH, Zen Y, Deshpande V. IgG4-related disease. N Engl J Med 2012;366(6):539-51.

Saeki T, Nishi S, Imai N, et al. Clinicopathological characteristics of patients with IgG4-related tubulointerstitial nephritis. Kidney Int 2010;78(10):1016-23.

NSAIDs and the kidney

De Broe ME, Elseviers MM. Analgesic nephropathy. N Engl J Med 1998;338(7):446-52.

Ejaz P, Bhojani K, Joshi VR. NSAIDs and kidney. J Assoc Physicians India. 2004; 52:632-40.

Huerta C, Castellsague J, Varas-Lorenzo C, Garcia Rodriguez LA. Nonsteroidal anti-inflammatory drugs and risk of ARF in the general population. Am J Kidney Dis 2005; 45(3):531-9.

Polycystic and other hereditary cystic kidney diseases

Rohatgi R. Clinical manifestations of hereditary cystic kidney disease. Front Biosci 2008;13:4175-97.

Torra Balcells R, Ars Criach E. Molecular diagnosis of autosomal dominant polycystic kidney disease. Nefrologia 2011;31:35-43.

Pei Y, Obaji J, Dupuis A, et al. Unified criteria for ultrasonographic diagnosis of ADPKD. J Am Soc Nephrol 2009;20:205-12.

Belibi FA, Edelstein CL. Unified ultrasonographic diagnostic criteria for polycystic kidney disease. J Am Soc Nephrol 2009;20:6-8.

Ravine D, Gibson RN, Walker RG, Sheffield LJ, Kincaid-Smith P, Danks DM. Evaluation of ultrasonographic diagnostic criteria for autosomal dominant polycystic kidney disease 1. Lancet 1994;343:824-7.

Kim I, Fu Y, Hui K, et al. Fibrocystin/polyductin modulates renal tubular formation by regulating polycystin-2 expression and function. J Am Soc Nephrol 2008;19:455-68.

Park EY, Woo YM, Park JH. Polycystic kidney disease and therapeutic approaches. BMB Rep 2011;44: 359-68.

Wuthrich RP, Serra AL, Kistler AD. Autosomal dominant polycystic kidney disease: new treatment options and how to test their efficacy. Kidney Blood Press Res 2009;32:380-7.

Torres VE, Boletta A, Chapman A, et al. Prospects for mTOR inhibitor use in patients with polycystic kidney disease and hamartomatous diseases. Clin J Am Soc Nephrol 2010;5:1312-29.

Takiar V, Nishio S, Seo-Mayer P, et al. Activating AMP-activated protein kinase (AMPK) slows renal cystogenesis. Proc Natl Acad Sci U S A 2011;108:2462-7.

Hildebrandt F, Otto E. Molecular genetics of nephronophthisis and medullary cystic kidney disease. J Am Soc Nephrol 2000;11:1753-61.

Katabathina VS, Kota G, Dasyam AK, et al. Adult renal cystic disease: a genetic, biological, and developmental primer. Radiographics 2010; 30(6):1509-23.

References and Suggested Reading

Obstructive uropathy

Tseng TY, Stoller ML. Obstructive uropathy. Clin Geriatr Med 2009; 25(3):437-43.

Riccabona M. Obstructive diseases of the urinary tract in children: lessons from the last 15 years. Pediatr Radiol 2010; 40(6):947-55.

Uppot RN. Emergent nephrostomy tube placement for acute urinary obstruction. Tech Vasc Interv Radiol 2009; 12(2):154-61.

Adamo R, Saad WE, Brown DB. Percutaneous ureteral interventions. Tech Vasc Interv Radiol 2009; 12(3):205-15.

Parsons BA, Hashim H. Emerging treatment options for benign prostatic obstruction. Curr Urol Rep 2011; 12(4):247-54.

Allen DJ, Longhorn SE, Philp T, et al. Percutaneous urinary drainage and ureteric stenting in malignant disease. Clin Oncol (R Coll Radiol) 2010; 22(9):733-9.

Urinary tract infection

Hooton TM, Stamm WE. Diagnosis and treatment of uncomplicated urinary tract infection. Infect Dis Clin North Am 1997;11(3):551-81.

Gupta K, Hooton TM, Naber KG, et al. International clinical practice guidelines for the treatment of acute uncomplicated cystitis and pyelonephritis in women: A 2010 update by the Infectious Diseases Society of America and the European Society for Microbiology and Infectious Diseases. Clin Infect Dis. 2011; 52:e103-20.

Heyns CF. Urinary tract infection associated with conditions causing urinary tract obstruction and stasis, excluding urolithiasis and neuropathic bladder. World J Urol 2012; 30(1):77-83.

9 Kidney Disorders in Other Diseases

9.1 Introduction

Kidneys may be involved in a variety of otherwise unrelated diseases. There are many potential mechanisms which may result in acute kidney injury, chronic kidney disease, electrolyte abnormalities, or acid-base disorders. Some of the kidney problems associated with underlying primary disease are described in other chapters. Here we will discuss kidney injury associated with diabetes mellitus, malignancies, hepatitis C, HIV infection, thrombotic microangiopathy, SLE, systemic sclerosis, and pregnancy.

9.2 Diabetic Nephropathy

Diabetic nephropathy is the leading cause of ESRD in the Western countries. In addition, diabetic renal disease increases the risk for cardiovascular mortality 20-40 fold. The risk of ESRD is now similar in type 1 and type 2 diabetes, and appears to be considerably reduced recently, to incidences under about 10% over 20 years, ascribed to improved management.

Stages of Diabetic Nephropathy			
	GFR	Albuminuria	Pathology
No nephropathy	Normal	None	Normal
Stage 1 and 2	Increased (hyperfiltration)	None	Glomerular hypertrophy
Stage 3: Initial diabetic nephropathy	Normal or decreased	Microalbuminuria (30 - 300 mg/d)	Thickening of the GBM, mesangial expansion, change in vascular cells, accumulation of advanced glycosylation end products
Advanced (overt) nephropathy	Declines by about 10ml/yr in untreated patients	Macroalbuminuria (>300 mg/d) and may have nephrotic syndrome	Kimmelstiel-Wilson nodules, increased glomerular basement membrane width, diffuse mesangial sclerosis, hyalinosis, microaneurysms, and hyaline arteriosclerosis, tubular and interstitial changes
ESRD	Very low	Heavy proteinuria	Advanced changes, including interstitial fibrosis and tubular atrophy

Risk Factors		
Risk factors for developing diabetic nephropathy	**Risk factors for progression of diabetic nephropathy**	**Risk factors for CV events**
• Glycemic control • Hypertension • Smoking • Cholesterol level • Advanced age • Insulin resistance • Male gender • Black, Hispanic, Asian, or Native American • Obesity • Family history of CV events • Genetic factors (eg, VEGF gene for retinopathy, the ELMO1 gene for nephropathy, and the ADIPOQ gene for coronary artery disease)	• Hypertension • Albuminuria • Glycemic control • Smoking	• Older age • Male gender • Longer duration of diabetes • CV disease history • Degree of albuminuria • Hypertension • Hypercholesterolemia

Diabetic Nephropathy: Treatment

Treatment

Goals
- Prevent progression of CKD
- Glycemic control
- Avoid cardiovascular events

Prevent progression of CKD
- Decreasing albuminuria is one goal of treatment
- ACEI or ARB due to renoprotective effect
- May potentially use ACEI+ARB combination in those with high risk for progression
- Blood pressure control (<130/80):
  Add antihypertensives as needed to ACEI or ARB
- Diet: Moderate protein reduction (0.7 to 0.9 g/kg body wt per d)
- Avoid nephrotoxic medications as much as possible

Glycemia control
- Poor glycemic control has been associated with increased microvascular complications
- Intensive glycemic control decreases nephropathy in type 1 and type 2 diabetics
- Role of intensive glycemic control:
  Does not reduce all-cause mortality, increases the risk of hypoglycemia by 30%, insufficient data to demonstrate reduction in cardiovascular mortality, composite microvascular complications, or retinopathy

CVD prophylaxis
- Blood pressure control
- Aspirin
- Treating dyslipidemia
- Beta-blockers when indicated

CKD Management of Diabetic Nephropathy
General management as in chapter on CKD with added attention to nutrition, hypercholesterolemia, sodium balance for better BP control, and avoidance of hyperkalemia (diabetic nephropathy is a common cause of type 4 RTA with hyperkalemia)
Control of general complications of CKD: anemia, hyperphosphatemia, hyperparathyroidism, and bone disease

9.3 Kidney Injury Associated with Malignancies

9.3.1 Kidney Dysfunction

Mechanical
- Extrarenal obstruction: Prostate, bladder, retroperitoneal or pelvic cancers
- Intrarenal tubular obstruction: Acute uric acid nephropathy, myeloma kidney (cast nephropathy)
- Tumor infiltration: Lymphoma or leukemia most commonly
- Renal ischemia: Renal vein occlusion from renal cell carcinoma

Hemodynamic alterations (hypovolemia, cardiac toxicity)

Glomerular diseases
- Membranous glomerulopathy (solid tumors)
- Minimal change nephropathy/FSGS (lymphomas and leukemias)
- Amyloidosis (myeloma, lymphoma, rarely leukemia or renal cell carcinoma)
- Membranoproliferative or rapidly progressive glomerulonephritis (solid tumors, lymphoma)
- Thrombotic microangiopathy: Some adenocarcinomas (pancreas, gastric)

Tubulointerstitial diseases
- Hypercalcemia: Acute renal failure, nephrogenic diabetes insipidus
- Multiple myeloma: Tubular dysfunction (see below)

9.3.2 Kidney dysfunction associated with the treatment of malignancies

- Radiation nephropathy or cystitis
- Complications of chemotherapy - renal failure
  - Hyperuricemia with urate nephropathy: "tumor lysis syndrome"
  - Cisplatin-, carboplatin-, and ifosfamide-induced acute renal failure
  - Interferon induced acute renal failure

- Complications of chemotherapy - renal failure (cont.)
  - HUS/TTP: Anti-tumor therapy (eg, mitomycin, bleomycin+cisplatin, gemcitabine, radiation+cyclophosphamide, vascular endothelial growth factor inhibitors)
  - High-dose methotrexate nephrotoxicity
  - High-dose bisphosphonate-induced acute renal failure or collapsing glomerulopathy
- Complications of chemotherapy - tubular disorders, bladder dysfunction
  - Tubular dysfunction: Hypokalemia, acidosis - ifosfamide, cisplatin
  - Hypomagnesemia: Cisplatin
  - Hemorrhagic cystitis: Cyclophosphamide, ifosfamide
  - Urinary retention: Vincristine

9.3.3   Electrolyte abnormalities associated with malignancies

- Vomiting and diarrhea: Hypokalemia, hyponatremia, acidosis or alkalosis
- Hyponatremia/SIADH: Tumor secretion of ADH, high dose cyclophosphamide, vincristine, vinblastine
- Hypercalcemia: Tumor secretion of PTH-RP, bone metastases, overproduction of 1,25 hydroxyvitamin D, cytokines
- Hyperphosphatemia, hyperkalemia, hypocalcemia with tumor lysis syndrome and ARF
- Hypokalemia: Lysozymuria with some leukemias
- Hypophosphatemia and tumor-induced osteomalacia: A rare syndrome characterized by urinary phosphate wasting, reduced 1,25-dihydroxyvitamin D concentrations, and osteomalacia.

9.3.4   Kidney disease in multiple myeloma

- Light chain toxicity
  - Myeloma kidney (ARF or CKD due to glomerular filtration of toxic light chains with tubular injury and obstruction - cast nephropathy)
  - Renal tubular dysfunction (accumulation of light chains in proximal cells causing Type 2 RTA or Fanconi syndrome - kappa chains more commonly)
- Amyloidosis - proteinuria or nephrotic syndrome, CKD (lambda chains more commonly)
- Cryoglobulinemia type 1 - membranoproliferative glomerular pattern - deposition of monoclonal immunoglobulin, usually IgG or IgM
- Hypercalcemia
- Hyperuricemia
- Increased risk for NSAID or radiocontrast nephrotoxicity
- Plasma cell renal infiltration

9.4   Kidney Disease in Hepatitis C

Hepatitis C can affect the kidneys by multiple mechanisms depicted below. There is evidence of direct viral invasion of the mesangium as well as immunological reaction that involves complement, immune complexes, antibodies against glomerular antigens, and cryoglobulins. The primary pathological presentation of hepatitis C associated glomerulonephritis is a membranoproliferative pattern.

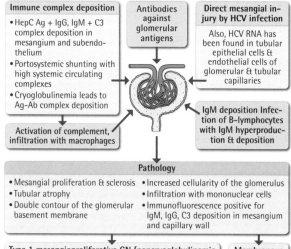

Immune complex deposition
- HepC Ag + IgG, IgM + C3 complex deposition in mesangium and subendothelium
- Portosystemic shunting with high systemic circulating complexes
- Cryoglobulinemia leads to Ag-Ab complex deposition

Antibodies against glomerular antigens

Direct mesangial injury by HCV infection

Also, HCV RNA has been found in tubular epithelial cells & endothelial cells of glomerular & tubular capillaries

Activation of complement, infiltration with macrophages

IgM deposition Infection of B-lymphocytes with IgM hyperproduction & deposition

Pathology
- Mesangial proliferation & sclerosis
- Tubular atrophy
- Double contour of the glomerular basement membrane
- Increased cellularity of the glomerulus
- Infiltration with mononuclear cells
- Immunofluorescence positive for IgM, IgG, C3 deposition in mesangium and capillary wall

Type 1 mesangioproliferative GN (noncryoglobulinemic & cryoglobulinemic), present with microscopic hematuria and proteinuria
- 50% present with mild-moderate renal insufficiency
- 20–25% present with acute nephritic syndrome
- 25% present with nephrotic syndrome

Membranous nephropathy
(80% present with nephrotic syndrome)

Treatment of Hepatitis C Associated Renal Disease
- Alfa interferon (3 million U TIW for 6-12 months SQ) or pegylated alfa interferon ± ribavirin
- Corticosteroids (may ameliorate renal dysfunction but may ↑ viremia and exacerbate hepatitis C)
- Plasmapheresis ± cytotoxic drugs for cryoglobulinemic MPGN

Cryoglobulinemia (may present with vasculitis/palpable purpura, arthralgias, lymphadenopathy, neuropathy, hepatosplenomegaly, hypocomplementemia, cryoglobulinemic nephropathy)

Type 1

Monoclonal immunoglobulin (multiple myeloma or Waldenstrom's macroglobulinemia)

Type 2

Essential mixed cryoglobulinemia - polyclonal immunoglobulins and a monoclonal IgM or IgG rheumatoid factor (infection with HCV or Epstein-Barr virus commonly)

Type 3

Mixed cryoglobulinemia - polyclonal IgGs and polyclonal IgMs (chronic inflammatory and autoimmune disorders: SLE, other connective tissue diseases, lymphoproliferative malignancies, HCV)

9.5   Human Immunodeficiency Virus (HIV) Infection

HIV infection can cause multiple renal injuries, including glomerular, interstitial, and/or tubular diseases. Furthermore, antiviral medications used in the treatment of HIV infection have possible adverse effects on the kidneys.

9.5.1   Kidney disease in HIV patients

Glomerular disease

- An immune complex glomerulonephritis with IgA deposits (IgA Ab against HIV)
- Membranoproliferative glomerulonephritis (associated with hepatitis C or mixed cryoglobulinemia due to HCV or HIV itself)
- FSGS (collapsing glomerulopathy with severe tubulointerstitial injury)
- Postinfectious glomerulonephritis
- Membranous nephropathy, due to concurrent infection with hepatitis B or C virus or syphilis
- Other immune complex kidney diseases (fibrillary GN, immunotactoid GN)

- Thrombotic microangiopathy (TTP/HUS)
- Crescentic GN: Lupus-like GN
- Pneumocystis jirovecii or Cryptococcus neoformans infection: Clumps of organisms obstructing glomerular and intertubular capillaries

Interstitial disease

- Viral: EBV, CMV, BK virus, direct infection by HIV, immune restoration inflammatory syndrome after initiation of HAART therapy
- Acute interstitial nephritis: β-lactam antibiotics, quinolones, trimethoprim-sulfa, rifampin
- Indinavir crystalluria

Acute tubular necrosis (ATN)

- Nephrotoxic medications: Pentamidine, foscarnet, cidofovir, adefovir, amphotericin B, aminoglycosides, trimethoprim-sulfa
- Intratubular obstruction (IV high-dose acyclovir or sulfadiazine)
- Infection/Sepsis
- Hypotension
- Rhabdomyolysis

9.5.2 Anti-HIV medications and kidney disorders

- ATN (pentamidine, foscarnet, cidofovir, amphotericin B, aminoglycosides, vancomycin, tenofovir, indinavir)
- Interstitial nephritis (TMP/SMX, NSAIDs, rifampin, beta-lactam antibiotics, ciprofloxacin and other quinolones, tenofovir, indinavir)
- Rhabdomyolysis (pentamidine, TMP/SMX, zidovudine, statins, tenofovir)
- Elevated creatinine (trimethoprim decreased tubular secretion of creatinine)
- Hyperkalemia (trimethoprim or pentamidine decreased tubular secretion of potassium)
- Hypokalemia (amphotericin B, didanosine, tenofovir)
- Hypocalcemia (pentamidine, foscarnet, didanosine)
- Hypomagnesemia (pentamidine, amphotericin B)
- Acidosis (amphotericin B, tenofovir)
- Diabetes insipidus, nephrogenic (foscarnet, tenofovir)
- Fanconi syndrome (tenofovir)
- Renal stones and nephropathy due to indinavir crystalluria

Risk Factors for Acute Renal Failure	
Risk factors specific to HIV	**Traditional risk factors**
• Male sex • CD4 cell count less than 200/μL • HIV RNA level greater than 10,000 copies/mL • Having ever received HAART • Hepatitis C coinfection	• Older age • Diabetes mellitus • Chronic kidney disease • Liver failure

9.6 Systemic Lupus Erythematosus (SLE)

SLE is one of the relatively common causes of kidney disease and renal failure. There are several pathological presentations of the SLE, which are summarized in the World Health Organization (WHO) classification below. Other classifications of SLE glomerular disease are very similar to the WHO classification of 1974: WHO morphologic classification of lupus nephritis (modified in 1982) and International Society of Nephrology/Renal Pathology Society (ISN/RPS) 2003 classification of lupus nephritis

9.6.1 World Health Organization (WHO) classification of lupus nephritis (1974)

Class	Pathology	Clinical Presentation	Treatment
I	No disease		
II	Mesangial GN	10–20% of cases; mildest, excellent prognosis: **IIa** - Just mesangial immune deposits **IIb** - Mesangial proliferation; mild proteinuria & hematuria	No therapy
III	Focal proliferative GN	10–20% of cases; prognosis is variable: Mild proteinuria & hematuria	Corticosteroids, immunosuppressives if severe, or no therapy if mild
IV	Diffuse proliferative GN	Most common and most severe: ARF/CKD, active lupus serology, active urinary sediment	Aggressive therapy: Corticosteroids + immunosuppressive therapy (cyclophosphamide or MMF or azathioprine

WHO classification of lupus nephritis (1974)			
Class	Pathology	Clinical Presentation	Treatment
V	Membranous glomerulopathy	10–20% of cases: Proteinuria or nephrotic syndrome	Sometimes not treated if asymptomatic, corticosteroids ± immunosuppressives (cyclophosphamide or cyclosporine or chlorambucil for severe nephrotic syndrome or progressive renal failure)
VI	Sclerosing	4% of cases: Represents healing of prior inflammatory injury	ACE inhibition
	Tubulointerstitial disease; vascular disease	Rare without glomerular disease	Corticosteroids

9.7 Thrombotic Microangiopathy (TMA)

9.7.1 Types

- Thrombotic thrombocytopenic purpura (TTP)
- Hemolytic uremic syndrome (HUS)

9.7.2 Causes

Thrombotic microangiopathy is caused by

- Underlying predisposing factors (eg, decreased C3 levels, decreased factor H, abnormal von Willebrand factor [vWF] cleaving protease activity or vWF gene mutation)
- Triggering events (eg, viruses, bacterial Shiga toxin/endotoxins, drugs, antibodies and immune complexes)
- The combination of the above two factors leads to loss of endothelial thromboresistance, leukocyte adhesion, vascular shear stress, consumption of complement, and abnormal vWF fragmentation

Thrombotic Microangiopathy

Thrombotic Microangiopathy
Occlusive microvascular thrombosis, hemolysis, thrombocytopenia, and end-organ damage

TTP
(Brain damage predominates)

Thrombocytopenia, hemolytic anemia, neurologic symptoms, renal functional abnormalities, fever (thrombi are rich in von Willebrand factor and platelets). Without treatment, mortality is up to 90%; relapses occur in over 1/3.

Congenital TTP
Deficiency of ADAMTS 13 (>50 mutations are described), a plasma metallo-protease that cleaves von Willebrand factor

Idiopathic TTP
Acquired deficiency of ADAMTS 13, e.g., due to antibody formation

Non-idiopathic TTP
Associated with
• Pregnancy
• Malignancy
• Drugs:
 - Cancer drugs: Mitomycin, cisplatin, gemcitabine, targeted cancer drugs;
 - Ticlopidine, clopidogrel
 - Quinine
 - Calcineurin inhibitors (cyclosporine, tacrolimus)
• Hematopoietic progenitor cell transplantation

Other causes of TMA
(Overlap with non-idiopathic TTP)
• Preeclampsia/HELLP
• Drugs
• Bone marrow or solid organ transplants
• Metastatic cancers
• Disseminated intravascular coagulopathy
• Lupus, rheumatoid arthritis, sclero derma, anti-phospholipid syndrome
• Infectious diseases (Rocky mountain spotted fever, anthrax)
• Intravascular devices (e.g., heart valves)
• Malignant HTN
• Cardiovascular procedures
• Paroxysmal nocturnal hemoglobinuria

HUS
• Renal damage predominates
• Thrombocytopenia, hemolytic anemia, renal failure (thrombi are rich in fibrin)
• Potentially high mortality especially among elderly; relapses much less common

Typical HUS: Diarrhea associated
Prodromal diarrheal illness caused by Shiga toxin-producing strain (e.g., E. Coli O157:H7 causes 95% of HUS in children, less common in adults)

Atypical HUS: Diarrhea negative
Relatively rare and hetero-geneous in etiology, e.g., mutation in complement regulation proteins, factor H, or factor B, activation of complement system: Low C3 and factor B

Treatment of HUS/TTP	
Plasma therapy – proven efficacy	**Medications**
• Plasma exchange (1-2 plasma volumes/day) • Plasma infusion • Plasma cryopheresis (for resistant forms) • Plasma exchange with solvent/detergent-treated plasma (for resistant forms, may limit the risk of viral contamination)	• Prednisone (commonly used) • Eculizumab for atypical HUS For poor responses: • IV gamma-globulin • Vincristine • Antithrombotic (heparin, tPA) and antiplatelet (aspirin) agents • Vitamin E

9.8 Systemic Sclerosis (SSc or scleroderma)

The pathogenesis of SSc includes vascular, immunological and fibrotic processes. It is characterized by fibrosis of the skin and visceral organs, and it has the highest mortality among connective tissue diseases (55% 10-year survival).

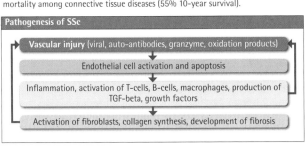

Pathogenesis of SSc

Vascular injury (viral, auto-antibodies, granzyme, oxidation products)

Endothelial cell activation and apoptosis

Inflammation, activation of T-cells, B-cells, macrophages, production of TGF-beta, growth factors

Activation of fibroblasts, collagen synthesis, development of fibrosis

Systemic Sclerosis: Types	
Limited cutaneous SSc	**Diffuse cutaneous SSc**
• Raynaud phenomenon • May have CREST syndrome (calcinosis cutis, Raynaud's, esophageal motility disorder, sclerodactyly, telangiectasia) • May have other organ involvement but less likely	• Raynaud phenomenon • Extracutaneous organ involvement more likely – Interstitial lung disease (earliest changes in the posterior lower lobes) – Pulmonary arterial hypertension (PAH) – Kidney injury and scleroderma renal crisis – Gastrointestinal involvement – Cardiac disease – Arthralgias, myalgias, contractures – Sexual dysfunction

9.8.1   Predictors of increased mortality

• Truncal skin involvement
• Abnormal ECG
• Reduced lung diffusing capacity
• Elevated ESR
• Presence of antibody to topoisomerase I (uncertain)

9.8.2   Scleroderma renal crisis

Occurs in 5-10% of SSc patients (15% of those with diffuse cutaneous SSc), caused by injury to medium-sized arteries in the kidneys and is a medical emergency.

Presentation
• Malignant hypertension with retinopathy • Encephalopathy and seizures • Hyperreninemia • Acute renal failure/RPGN • Proteinuria • Pulmonary edema • Headaches, fevers, malaise. • Normotensive scleroderma renal crisis is associated with a worse outcome

Patients at greatest risk for severe consequences
• Diffuse cutaneous or rapidly progressive forms of SSc
• Large joint contractures and tendon friction rubs
• Anemia
• New cardiac events
• Recent treatment with high-dose corticosteroids (≥15 mg prednisone/day)
• Positive ANA with speckled pattern
• Antibodies to RNA polymerase III
• Absence of anti-centromere antibodies.

Laboratory tests
Elevated creatinine, proteinuria/glomerulonephritis, microangiopathic hemolytic anemia, thrombocytopenia, hyperreninemia.

Treatment
• ACEI (particularly captopril)
• Role of ARB is unknown
• Endothelin might be a potential target
• 40% may require dialysis

9.9 Pregnancy

Consulting on pregnant patients may be an important part of some nephrology practices. Three common issues that trigger consultations are: **diminished renal function, proteinuria, and hypertension** as signs of either a non-pregnancy-related condition or preeclampsia. When measuring kidney function, it is important to realize that formulae used to estimate GFR (eg, Cockcroft-Gault, MDRD formula) are inaccurate, and a measured creatinine clearance based on a timed urine collection (usually 24 hr) remains the most practical. Similarly, to quantitate proteinuria, the protein-to-crea-tinine ratio can be used to monitor changes in the amount of proteinuria over time, but to determine the absolute value of proteinuria over 24 hours, it is best to measure in a 24-hr collection.

Proteinuria In Pregnancy		
Normal	**Kidney disease:**	**Preeclampsia**
• <200-300 of protein/24 h (secondary to ↑ GFR, ↑ basement membrane permeability)	Pregnancy may • Unmask kidney disease • Worsen preexisting kidney disease • Be a time in which de novo renal disease develops	Signs are • Hypertension • Proteinuria • Edema • Multiorgan injury, eg, kidney, CNS, liver, thrombotic microangiopathy

9.9.1   Causes of high blood pressure in pregnancy

- Chronic essential HTN
- Secondary hypertension
- Preeclampsia
- Preeclampsia superimposed on chronic HTN
- Gestational HTN

9.9.2   Causes of ARF in pregnancy

- Prerenal causes of ischemia, cardiomyopathy
- Thrombotic microangiopathies (preeclampsia, HELLP syndrome, acute fatty liver of pregnancy, TTP)
- Acute tubular necrosis
- Renal cortical necrosis
- Postpartum acute renal failure
- Obstructive uropathy, nephrolithiasis
- Acute pyelonephritis

9.9.3   Treatment of preeclampsia

MgSO4 parenterally most common – serum therapeutic level 4–6 mg/dL (follow hyperreflexia) in moderate or severe preeclampsia to prophylax for seizures (eclampsia)

Rx of HTN:

- If BP <140/90, protein <500 mg/24 h - mild disease → close follow-up, reduced activity, fetal assessments
- If BP ≥140/95, decreased renal function, increased uric acid, proteinuria >500 mg/24 h → hospitalization and delivery if >32-34 weeks, gestation; if possible, lower BP to 140/90 before delivery with antihypertensives tolerated in pregnancy, eg, calcium channel blockers, beta-blockers, hydralazine, methyldopa. If <32 weeks, close observation with maternal and fetal monitoring, BP control, seizure (eclampsia) prevention (IV MgSO4), and corticosteroids for fetal lung maturation in an attempt to keep the patient stable to improve fetal viability, but if symptoms/signs worsen, delivery may become necessary.
- If BP >160/100 - parenteral Rx (labetalol, hydralazine, nicardipine) → urgent delivery if seizure (eclampsia), severe renal failure or HELLP syndrome develops.

9.10   Important Inherited Disorders

Inherited Disorders	Extrarenal Manifestations	Renal Manifestations
Hereditary nephritis (Alport syndrome)	Hearing loss, ocular disease, hypertension, leiomyomatosis	Microhematuria, proteinuria, progressive CKD, renal pathology of split or laminated GBM on EM and absence of anti-GBM Ab staining on immunofluorecsence due to genetic defects in Type IV collagen
Von Hippel–Lindau disease	Retinal lesions (angiomas), cerebral hemangioma, pheochromocytoma, pancreatic cystadenomas and neuroendocrine tumors	Renal hemangioblastomas, renal cell carcinomas (up to 70%)
Tuberous sclerosis	Seizures, multiorgan tumors, cardiac rhabdomyomas, retinal hamartomas/angiofibromas, pulmonary lymphangioleiomyomatosis (LAM)	Renal angiomyolipomas, multiple cysts, renal hemorrhages, renal cell carcinomas (1-2%), may benefit from eculizumab treatment
Beckwith–Wiedemann syndrome	Visceromegaly, macroglossia, abdominal wall defect, prenatal and postnatal overgrowth, neonatal hypoglycemia, abdominal organ neoplasms	Wilms' tumor, medullary dysplasia, hypercalciuria, nephrolithiasis
Retinitis pigmentosa	Retinitis pigmentosa	Nephronophthisis (small hyperechoic kidneys with smooth outline cysts), chronic tubulointerstitial disease, renal sodium wasting, CKD

Polycystic kidney disease is included in the chapter on interstitial, cystic, infectious, and obstructive diseases.

References and Suggested Reading

Kidney Disorders in Diabetes Mellitus

Abaterusso C, Lupo A, Ortalda V, et al. Treating elderly people with diabetes and stages 3 and 4 chronic kidney disease. Clin J Am Soc Nephrol 2008;3:1185-94.

Remuzzi G, Macia M, Ruggenenti P. Prevention and treatment of diabetic renal disease in type 2 diabetes: the BENEDICT study. J Am Soc Nephrol 2006;17:S90-7.

Berl T, Hunsicker LG, Lewis JB, et al. Cardiovascular outcomes in the Irbesartan Diabetic Nephropathy Trial of patients with type 2 diabetes and overt nephropathy. Ann Intern Med 2003;138:542-9.

Vejakama P, Thakkinstian A, Lertrattananon D, et al. Reno-protective effects of renin-angiotensin system blockade in type 2 diabetic patients: a systematic review and network meta-analysis. Diabetologia 2011;55:566-78.

Effect of intensive therapy on the development and progression of diabetic nephropathy in the Diabetes Control and Complications Trial. The Diabetes Control and Complications (DCCT) Research Group. Kidney Int 1995;47:1703-20.

Reichard P, Nilsson BY, Rosenqvist U. The effect of long-term intensified insulin treatment on the development of microvascular complications of diabetes mellitus. N Engl J Med 1993;329:304-9.

Pichler RH, de Boer IH. Dual renin-angiotensin-aldosterone system blockade for diabetic kidney disease. Curr Diab Rep 2010;10:297-305.

Bash LD, Selvin E, Steffes M, et al. Poor glycemic control in diabetes and the risk of incident chronic kidney disease even in the absence of albuminuria and retinopathy: Atherosclerosis Risk in Communities (ARIC) Study. Arch Intern Med 2008;168:2440-7.

Hemmingsen B, Lund SS, Gluud C, et al. Targeting intensive glycaemic control versus targeting conventional glycaemic control for type 2 diabetes mellitus. Cochrane Database Syst Rev 2011:CD008143.

Patel A, MacMahon S, Chalmers J, et al. Intensive blood glucose control and vascular outcomes in patients with type 2 diabetes. N Engl J Med 2008;358:2560-72.

KDOQI clinical practice guidelines and clinical practice recommendations for diabetes and chronic kidney disease. Am J Kidney Dis 2007;49:S1-S179.

Doria A. Genetics of diabetes complications. Curr Diab Rep 2010;10:467-75.

Hemmingsen B, Lund SS, Gluud C, et al. Intensive glycaemic control for patients with type 2 diabetes: systematic review with meta-analysis and trial sequential analysis of randomised clinical trials. BMJ 2011;343:d6898.

Fioretto P, Mauer M. Reversal of diabetic nephropathy: lessons from pancreas transplantation. J Nephrol 2012;25:13-8.

Kidney Disorders in Malignancy

Buemi M, Fazio MR, Bolignano D, et al. Renal complications in oncohematologic patients. J Investig Med 2009; 57(8):892-901.

Skinner R. Nephrotoxicity--what do we know and what don't we know? J Pediatr Hematol Oncol 2011; 33(2):128-34.

Cairo MS, Coiffier B, Reiter A, Younes A. Recommendations for the evaluation of risk and prophylaxis of tumour lysis syndrome (TLS) in adults and children with malignant diseases: an expert TLS panel consensus. Br J Haematol 2010; 149(4):578-86.

Gurevich F, Perazella MA. Renal effects of anti-angiogenesis therapy: update for the internist. Am J Med 2009; 122(4):322-8.

Humphreys BD, Soiffer RJ, Magee CC. Renal failure associated with cancer and its treatment: an update. J Am Soc Nephrol 2005;16(1):151-61.

Chong WH, Molinolo AA, Chen CC, Collins MT. Tumor-induced osteomalacia. Endocr Relat Cancer. Jun 2011;18(3): R53-77.

References and Suggested Reading (cont.)

Kidney Disorders in Hepatitis C

Fabrizi F, Martin P, Dixit V, Messa P. Hepatitis C virus infection and kidney disease: a meta-analysis. Clin J Am Soc Nephrol 2012; 7(4):549-57.

Perico N, Cattaneo D, Bikbov B, Remuzzi G. Hepatitis C infection and chronic renal diseases. Clin J Am Soc Nephrol 2009;4:207-20.

Praga M, GutiÀrrez SolÀs E, Morales E. Hepatitis C-induced renal disease in patients with AIDS: an emergent problem. Contrib Nephrol 2012; 176:24-34.

Martin P, Fabrizi F. Hepatitis C virus and kidney disease. J Hepatol 2008; 49(4):613-24.

Kidney Disorders in HIV

Maggi P, Bartolozzi D, Bonfanti P, et al. Renal complications in HIV disease: between present and future. AIDS Rev 2012; 14(1):37-53.

Wyatt CM, Meliambro K, Klotman PE. Recent progress in HIV-associated nephropathy. Annu Rev Med 2012; 63:147-59

Atta MG. Diagnosis and natural history of HIV-associated nephropathy. Adv Chronic Kidney Dis 2010; 17(1):52-8.

Cooper RD, Tonelli M. Renal disease associated with antiretroviral therapy in the treatment of HIV. Nephron Clin Pract 2011; 118(3):c262-8.

Elewa U, Sandri AM, Rizza SA, Fervenza FC. Treatment of HIV-associated nephropathies. Nephron Clin Pract 2011; 118(4):c346-54; discussion c354.

Hall AM, Hendry BM, Nitsch D, Connolly JO. Tenofovir-associated kidney toxicity in HIV-infected patients: a review of the evidence. Am J Kidney Dis 2011; 57(5):773-80.

Wyatt CM, Malvestutto C, Coca SG, Klotman PE, Parikh CR. The impact of hepatitis C virus coinfection on HIV-related kidney disease: a systematic review and meta-analysis. AIDS 2008; 22(14):1799-807.

Kidney Disorders in SLE

Weening JJ, D'Agati VD, Schwartz MM, et al. The classification of glomerulonephritis in systemic lupus erythematosus revisited. J Am Soc Nephrol 2004;15:241-50.

Tsokos GC. Systemic lupus erythematosus. N Engl J Med 2011; 365(22):2110-21.

Alshayeb H, Wall BM, Gosmanova EO. Treatment of proliferative and membranous lupus nephritis: review of key clinical trials. Am J Med Sci 2013; 343(1):86-90.

Appel GB. New and future therapies for lupus nephritis. Cleve Clin J Med 2012; 79(2):134-40.

Shum K, Askanase A. Treatment of lupus nephritis. Curr Rheumatol Rep 2011; 13(4):283-90.

Swan JT, Riche DM, Riche KD, Majithia V. Systematic review and meta-analysis of immunosuppressant therapy clinical trials in membranous lupus nephritis. J Investig Med 2011; 59(2):246-58.

Lee YH, Lee HS, Choi SJ, et al. Efficacy and safety of tacrolimus therapy for lupus nephritis: a systematic review of clinical trials. Lupus 2011; 20(6):636-40.

Kamanamool N, McEvoy M, Attia J, et al. Efficacy and adverse events of mycophenolate mofetil versus cyclophosphamide for induction therapy of lupus nephritis: systematic review and meta-analysis. Medicine (Baltimore) 2010; 89(4):227-35.

Hogan J, Schwenk MH, Radhakrishnan J. Should mycophenolate mofetil replace cyclophosphamide as first-line therapy for severe lupus nephritis? Kidney Int 2012; 82(12):1256-60.

References and Suggested Reading (cont.)

Ramos-Casals M, Diaz-Lagares C, Soto-Cardenas MJ, et al. Rituximab therapy in lupus nephritis: current clinical evidence. Clin Rev Allergy Immunol 2011; 40(3):159-69.

Mok CC, Cheung TT, Lo WH. Minimal mesangial lupus nephritis: a systematic review. Scand J Rheumatol 2010; 39(3): 181-9.

Smyth A, Oliveira GH, Lahr BD, et al. A systematic review and meta-analysis of pregnancy outcomes in patients with systemic lupus erythematosus and lupus nephritis. Clin J Am Soc Nephrol 2010; 5(11): 2060-8.

Kidney Disorders in Thrombotic Microangiopathies (TTP and HUS)

Ruggenenti P, Noris M, Remuzzi G. Thrombotic microangiopathy, hemolytic uremic syndrome, and thrombotic thrombocytopenic purpura. Kidney Int 2001;60:831-46.

Tsai HM. Advances in the pathogenesis, diagnosis, and treatment of thrombotic thrombocytopenic purpura. J Am Soc Nephrol 2003;14:1072-81.

Blake-Haskins JA, Lechleider RJ, Kreitman RJ. Thrombotic microangiopathy with targeted cancer agents. Clin Cancer Res 2011;17:5858-66.

Zheng XL, Sadler JE. Pathogenesis of thrombotic microangiopathies. Annu Rev Pathol 2008;3:249-77.

Desch K, Motto D. Is there a shared pathophysiology for thrombotic thrombocytopenic purpura and hemolytic-uremic syndrome? J Am Soc Nephrol 2007;18:2457-60.

Tsai HM. The molecular biology of thrombotic microangiopathy. Kidney Int 2006;70:16-23.

Schmidtko J, Peine S, El-Housseini Y, et al. Treatment of atypical hemolytic uremic syndrome and thrombotic microangiopathies: a focus on eculizumab. Am J Kidney Dis 2013; 61(2):289-99.

Kidney Disorders in Systemic Sclerosis (Scleroderma)

Varga J. Systemic sclerosis: an update. Bull NYU Hosp Jt Dis 2008;66:198-202.

Denton CP. Renal manifestations of systemic sclerosis--clinical features and outcome assessment. Rheumatology (Oxford) 2008;47 Suppl 5:v54-6.

Denton CP, Lapadula G, Mouthon L, Muller-Ladner U. Renal complications and scleroderma renal crisis. Rheumatology (Oxford) 2009;48 Suppl 3:iii32-5.

Lim IG, Schrieber L. Management of systemic sclerosis. Isr Med Assoc J 2002;4:953-7.

Kidney Disorders in Pregnancy

Maynard SE, Thadhani R. Pregnancy and the kidney. J Am Soc Nephrol 2009;20:14-22.

Ganesan C, Maynard SE. Acute kidney injury in pregnancy: the thrombotic microangiopathies. J Nephrol 2011;24:554-63.

Podymow T, August P, Akbari A. Management of renal disease in pregnancy. Obstet Gynecol Clin North Am 2010; 37(2):195-21.

Mirza FG, Cleary KL. Pre-eclampsia and the kidney. Semin Perinatol 2009; 33(3):173-8.

Stillman IE, Karumanchi SA. The glomerular injury of preeclampsia. J Am Soc Nephrol 2007; 18(8):2281-4.

Baumwell S, Karumanchi SA. Pre-eclampsia: clinical manifestations and molecular mechanisms. Nephron Clin Pract 2007; 106(2):c72-81.

Fischer MJ. Chronic kidney disease and pregnancy: maternal and fetal outcomes. Adv Chronic Kidney Dis 2007; 14(2):132-45.

Krane NK, Hamrahian M. Pregnancy: kidney diseases and hypertension. Am J Kidney Dis 2007; 49(2): 336-45.

References and Suggested Reading (cont.)

Kidney Disorders in Hereditary Diseases

Kashtan CE. Alport syndrome. An inherited disorder of renal, ocular, and cochlear basement membranes. Medicine (Baltimore) 1999; 78(5):338-60.

Lonser RR, Glenn GM, Walther M, et al. von Hippel-Lindau disease. Lancet 2003; 361(9374):2059-67.

Curatolo P, Bombardieri R, Jozwiak S. Tuberous sclerosis. Lancet 2008; 372(9639):657-68.

Enklaar T, Zabel BU, Prawitt D. Beckwith-Wiedemann syndrome: multiple molecular mechanisms. Expert Rev Mol Med 2006; 8(17):1-19.

Bissler JJ, Kingswood JC, Radzikowska E, at al. "Everolimus for angiomyolipoma associated with tuberous sclerosis complex or sporadic lymphangioleiomyomatosis (EXIST-2): a multicentre, randomised, double-blind, placebo-controlled trial. The Lancet, 11 January 2013; doi:10.1016/S0140-6736(12)61767-X

Caridi G, Dagnino M, Gusmano R, et al. Clinical and molecular heterogeneity of juvenile nephronophthisis in Italy: insights from molecular screening. Am J Kidney Dis 2000; 35(1):44-51.

Otto EA, Hurd TW, Airik R, et al. Candidate exome capture identifies mutation of SDCCAG8 as the cause of a retinal-renal ciliopathy. Nat Genet 2010; 42(10):840-50.

10　Hypertension & RAS

10.1　Staging of Hypertension (HTN)

Staging of Hypertension (According to JNC-7) *		
BP Value	**Stage**	**Treatment**
<120/80	Normal	–
120-139/80-89	Prehypertension	Does not require drugs, but early interventions of lifestyle modifications (weight loss, low salt and/or DASH diet, increased physical activity, and limiting alcohol) could reduce BP and delay/prevent the onset of HTN
140-159/90-99	HTN stage 1	Treatment is indicated: Usually start with one antihypertensive drug
≥160/≥100	HTN stage 2	May start with two drugs

* The Seventh Report of the Joint National Committee on Prevention, Detection, Evaluation, and Treatment of High Blood Pressure. August, 2004. http://www.nhlbi.nih.gov/guidelines/hypertension/jnc7full.pdf. Accessed October 8, 2012
* Chobanian AV, Bakris GL, Black HR, et al. The Seventh Report of the Joint National Committee on Prevention, Detection, Evaluation, and Treatment of High Blood Pressure: the JNC 7 report. JAMA 2003;289:2560-72.

10.2　Classification of HTN

Classification	Definition	Treatment
Resistant HTN	BP ≥ 140/90 despite 3 drug Rx including a diuretic	Evaluate for causes and adherence to therapy (see below), lifestyle modifications as listed above, consider ambulatory BP monitoring
Refractory HTN	BP ≥ 140/90 despite ≥ 4 drug Rx at maximal doses	Same as resistant HTN plus sympatholytic Rx may be effective in this group; renal sympathetic denervation and carotid sinus stimulation are investigational treatments
HTN urgency	Asymptomatic BP ≥ 180-200/120	BP control to 140/90 over several days

Classification	Definition	Treatment
HTN emergency (accelerated or malignant HTN)	Symptomatic with retinal hemorrhages, papilledema, neurologic symptoms, encephalopathy, and/or malignant nephrosclerosis; BP ≥180-200/120 (usually but not required)	Hospitalization and parenteral Rx (see below) to reduce diastolic BP to 100-110 in several hours then gradual reduction to 80-90 over several weeks; overly aggressive reduction in BP may cause coronary, cerebral, or renal ischemia; evaluate for secondary causes of HTN
HTN in pregnancy	BP ≥140/ ≥90 but must differentiate: • Chronic essential HTN (presenting at <20 wks) • Preeclampsia (new onset >20 wks but may be superimposed on chronic HTN) • Transient (gestational) HTN near term	Treatment is indicated if BP >150/ >100, end-organ damage, or preeclampsia (see Rx below and chapter "Kidney Disorders in Other Diseases")

Which blood pressure reading should be followed?

- **Systolic blood pressure** has a better association with CVD risk than diastolic in those older than 50; in younger patients, diastolic BP is a better predictor.
- **24-hour blood pressure monitoring** is the gold standard, otherwise office BP may be used; home BP is reliable but both tend to lead to overdiagnosis.
- Consider **ambulatory BP monitoring** to evaluate the circadian rhythm of BP readings (eg, higher values while awake; lower values at nighttime - BP "dipping"); control of nighttime, rather than daytime, BP seems most associated with better outcomes
- **Goal** BP ≤ 140/90 mmHg unless patient has diabetes mellitus or kidney disease when goal BP ≤ 130-135/80-85 mmHg

10.3   Causes of Resistant or Refractory HTN

- Secondary HTN (see below)
- Improper BP measurements or "white-coat" HTN
- Calcification or sclerosis of brachial arteries (falsely high by arm sphygmomano-me-ter)
- Nonadherence to anti-HTN medications
- Use of other drugs (over-the-counter meds, eg, NSAIDs, decongestants)
- Dietary indiscretion of salt or alcohol
- Volume overload with inadequate diuretic therapy
- Comorbidities (eg, obesity, obstructive sleep apnea)

10.4   Evaluation of Secondary Causes of Hypertension

Evaluation of Secondary Causes of Hypertension especially in young onset, resistant or accelerated HTN.

Patient Studies
• History: HTN related to drugs - hormonal contraceptives, NSAIDs, cocaine, amphetamines, sympathomimetics, corticosteroids, licorice, epoetin, excessive alcohol
• Endocrinopathies: Hyperthyroidism, Cushing's syndrome, pheochromocytoma
• Sleep study if obstructive sleep apnea is considered
• Ambulatory 24-hr BP monitoring ("white coat" labile hypertension, nighttime dipping)

Laboratory Tests
All patients
• Creatinine (renal function)
• Urinalysis (detect proteinuria, kidney disease)
• Electrolytes/glucose (hypokalemia, metabolic alkalosis, or diabetes may suggest hypermineralocorticoid state)
Specific studies (based on findings)
• Aldosterone, renin levels (primary hyperaldosteronism or secondary hyperreninemic state, eg, renal artery stenosis, kidney tumor)
• TSH (hyperthyroidism)
• Cortisol (Cushing's syndrome)
• Plasma or urine catecholamines (pheochromocytoma)
• Drug screening (eg, cocaine)

Radiologic Imaging
• Renal ultrasound with Doppler (cystic/anatomic diseases, obstructive uropathy, signs of renal artery stenosis) • CT or MR angiogram (detect/confirm renal artery stenosis, fibromuscular dysplasia, coarctation of the aorta) • Radiocontrast angiography (confirm main or segmental renal artery stenosis) • Adrenal vein aldosterone and cortisol levels for laterality of adrenal adenomas

10.5 Evaluation of End-Organ Damage Secondary to HTN

Microvascular	Macrovascular	Cardiac
• Retinopathy • Nephropathy • Encephalopathy	• Coronary artery disease • Cerebrovascular disease/stroke • Peripheral arterial disease • Aortic dissection	• Myocardial remodeling and LVH • Congestive heart failure

10.6 Selection of Initial Therapy

Selection of Initial Therapy in Patients with No Specific Indications
Stage 1: Diuretic or angiotensin converting enzyme inhibitor (ACEI) or angiotensin receptor blocker (ARB) or beta-blocker (BB), or calcium channel blocker (CCB)
Stage 2: Diuretic AND ACEI or ARB or BB or CCB

Selection of Initial Therapy Based on Demographics
• In Blacks, ACEI may be less effective in lowering blood pressure than either thiazide-type diuretic or CCB. • Blacks and Asians have greater rates of angioedema and cough as side effects with ACEI. • In elderly patients, HTN and isolated systolic HTN should be treated; thiazides with or without amiloride, ACEI, BB, and long-acting CCB have been shown beneficial; alpha blockers should be avoided due to adverse effects unless indicated for symptoms of prostatic hypertrophy

10.7 Treatment

Treatment Based on Specific Indications or Comorbid Conditions

Patients with kidney disease

- In patients with proteinuric renal disease: ACEI or ARB may slow progression of CKD; combining ACEI and ARB together may decrease proteinuria further, but at the expense of greater side effects and ACEI + ARB combinations are probably best avoided in older patients. Aliskiren has been shown to decrease proteinuria, but long-term effect on CKD needs elucidation
- With chronic renal failure: Diuretics are a primary therapeutic modality (thiazides or loop diuretics) to achieve BP control by relieving hypervolemia
- In CKD patients: ≥ 3 drugs including a diuretic are commonly needed to achieve goal BP ≤ 135/85

Patients with diabetes mellitus

- With proteinuria: ACEI or ARB first to slow progression of CKD, low-dose diuretic, CCB as needed to achieve goal BP £ 130/80
- Thiazide diuretics may worsen glucose tolerance: Potassium depletion may impair pancreatic islet beta-cell insulin release and thiazides may increase insulin resistance of target tissues (avoid by potassium repletion, use low-dose with co-administration of ACEI or ARB).
- Beta-blockers may have deleterious metabolic consequences: Increased severity and duration of hypoglycemic episodes in Type 1 DM by impairing the hepatic glycogenolytic response to adrenal epinephrine release in hypoglycemia (decrease this effect by using cardioselective beta-blockers at low dose). Beta-blockers may elevate plasma triglycerides (beta-blockers with intrinsic sympathomimetic (partial agonist) activity (e.g. pindolol or acebutolol) are less likely to cause this effect)

Patients with resistant or refractory HTN

- Low sodium diet should be stressed (test for 24 hr urinary Na excretion)
- Diuretics (counter the volume expansion caused by other anti-HTN agents and potentiate their effect). Start with thiazides, use loop diuretics in those with low GFR, and consider adding aldosterone blockade with spironolactone or eplerenone or potassium-sparing collecting-duct sodium channel blockade with amiloride
- Combine effects of different anti-HTN medication classes: Renin-angiotensin-aldosterone antagonism with ACEI, ARB or aliskiren, BB (eg, labetalol or carvedilol), long-acting CCB, CNS acting agent (eg, clonidine), direct vasodilator (eg, hydralazine or minoxidil)
- Consider investigational use of endovascular radiofrequency renal sympathetic denervation or electrical stimulation of carotid sinus baroreceptors in severe cases

Treatment Based on Specific Indications or Comorbid Conditions

Patients with HTN emergency (accelerated or malignant HTN)

- Start with parenteral IV administration: Commonly either a direct vasodilator (nitroprusside) or an alpha & beta sympatholytic (labetalol) or a CCB with vasodilator activity (nicardipine or clevidipine) or a postsynaptic dopamine receptor agonist (fenoldopam)
- Other IV medications that can be used: Esmolol, enalaprilat, hydralazine, urapidil
- Loop diuretic for volume overload
- Follow with oral agents as for resistant HTN, combining effects of different classes, eg, captopril, labetalol, amiloride, clonidine, prazosin, hydralazine

Patients with CHF and ischemic heart disease

- ACEI or ARB as initial therapy for CHF
- Beta-blockers (eg, carvedilol) as initial therapy for ischemic heart disease
- Diuretics (for peripheral or pulmonary edema)
- Aldosterone antagonists (spironolactone or eplerenone)
- Long-acting CCB if needed
- Direct vasodilators (eg, hydralazine) may be considered for CHF if necessary, but are not advised in patients with LVH

Patients with sleep apnea

- Nasal continuous positive airway pressure may be effective treatment of HTN
- Weight reduction for obesity
- Otherwise conventional antihypertensive treatment should be undertaken

Patients with obstructive airways disease (COPD or asthma)

- Beta-adrenergic antagonists should be considered second-line therapy, unless there is another indication (eg, coronary artery disease), in which case selective beta-1-blocker should be preferred

Patients with dyslipidemia

- Thiazides may increase serum cholesterol levels, especially LDL, however the effect is generally dose dependent; co-administration of an ACEI blunts or abolishes thiazide-induced metabolic abnormalities
- Beta-blockers cause an elevation in serum triglyceride levels (beta-blockers with intrinsic sympathomimetic (partial agonist) activity (e.g. pindolol or acebutolol) are less likely to cause this effect).
- ACE inhibitors and calcium channel antagonists have little effect on lipids
- Alpha-1-antagonists may elevate HDL

Treatment Based On Specific Indications Or Comorbid Conditions

Pregnant patients

- Methyldopa, hydralazine - long-term safety data
- Long-acting CCB
- Beta-blockers - generally safe, but may impair fetal growth when used early (atenolol)
- Diuretics controversial - okay for volume overload
- Acute treatment - parenteral labetalol, hydralazine or nicardipine
- ACEI, nitroprusside - **contraindicated** in pregnancy

Patients with pheochromocytoma

- Preoperative management: alpha-adrenergic blockade (eg, oral phenoxybenza-mine for control of BP and tachyarrhythmias).
- If alpha-blockade alone does not normalize BP and HR, beta-blockers may be added (eg, propranolol) to control BP and HR. Beta-blockade may be used only after effective alpha-blockade is in place to prevent unopposed alpha-adrenergically mediated vasoconstriction by elevated circulating catecholamines.
- Preoperative management should include intravascular volume expansion: Some patients with pheochromocytoma are volume-contracted

Patients with other conditions

- Atrial fibrillation: Beta-blockers help control heart rate
- Essential tremor: Beta-blockers have beneficial effect on tremor
- Prostatic hypertrophy: Alpha-blockers help voiding hesitancy
- Obese patients: weight reduction is a primary goal of Rx
- Scleroderma (progressive systemic sclerosis): ACEI is preferred therapy, with cap-topril used most commonly, or an ARB if ACEI isn't tolerated; CCB or a direct vaso-dilator added if necessary; BB may aggravate Raynaud phenomenon so should be avoided

10.8   Renal Artery Stenosis (RAS)

10.8.1   Causes of RAS

- Atherosclerosis (most common - 90% of cases)
- Fibromuscular dysplasia
- Other: Vasculitis, neurofibromatosis, congenital bands, extrinsic compression, and radiation.

10.8.2 Evaluation of patient for RAS

- Renal ultrasound with Doppler detects RAS with ~ 80% sensitivity.
- Ultrasound resistive indices are helpful to predict outcome of intervention (better when < 80; poorer when >80)
- Radiocontrast CT angiography
- MR angiography
- Radiocontrast aortography and selective renal arteriography (to confirm RAS, particularly for segmental or fibromuscular arterial disease)
- Renal vein renin levels to assess lateralization when findings are indecisive (false positives and negatives have decreased this test's usefulness)
- Radionuclide renography to assess differential renal blood flow and function (as a percentage of overall renal function)

10.8.3 Treatment of RAS

Medical therapy

- ACEI or ARB is effective in >85% of patients but has risk of a hemodynamic decrease in renal function, particularly with bilateral RAS
- Often need to combine Rx with a diuretic
- Should urge smoking cessation, lipid-lowering Rx, and aspirin or anti-platelet agents, if indicated

Interventional therapy

Revascularization is not indicated in all patients since overall results are similar to medical Rx; should be considered in those with hemodynamically significant RAS with worsening renal function, difficult to control hypertension, unexplained flash pulmonary edema, or perhaps unstable angina.

- Percutaneous intervention: Balloon angioplasty, with or without stenting is treatment of choice for patients with fibromuscular dysplasia, less effective for atherosclerotic RAS due to potential for intimal dissection, elastic recoil and rigidity of the lesions, and atheroemboli.
- Randomized trials indicate that the procedure is less effective in controlling blood pressure and renal function than in reducing BP medications.
- Treatment with aspirin before the procedure and the use of an iso-osmolar contrast medium and heparin during the procedure may improve the success rate to > 80% with a recurrence rate of 10%
- Surgical revascularization may be indicated for certain cases not amenable to percutaneous angioplasty: Unilateral aortorenal bypass surgery and extra-anatomical bypass (bypass originates from the celiac or mesenteric branches). Perioperative mortality rates range from > 2% for aortorenal procedures to > 6% for extra-anatomical vascular bypasses

10.9   Hypertensive Nephropathy

Hypertensive Nephropathy/Hypertensive Nephrosclerosis

Hypertensive nephropathy is thought to be the second most common cause of ESRD after diabetic nephropathy. If HTN is poorly controlled, renal insufficiency may progress slowly over years with "benign nephrosclerosis", the nephropathy associated with "benign hypertension" whereas with malignant hypertension, "malignant nephrosclerosis" is a rapidly progressive renal disease with ESRD that may occur in weeks.

10.9.1   Predictors of kidney injury

- Severity of HTN
- Presence of comorbid conditions (eg, diabetes)
- Male gender
- African American race (a co-existing condition of genetic focal segmental glomerular sclerosis may be a contributing cause of progressive nephropathy - see chapter on Glomerular Diseases)

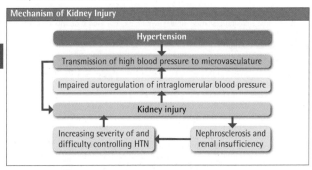

Mechanism of Kidney Injury

Hypertension

Transmission of high blood pressure to microvasculature

Impaired autoregulation of intraglomerular blood pressure

Kidney injury

Increasing severity of and difficulty controlling HTN ← Nephrosclerosis and renal insufficiency

10.9.2   Clinical manifestations

- Proteinuria
- Renal insufficiency
- Hematuria (usually with malignant hypertension)
- Possible association with other hypertensive end-organ damage (hypertensive retinopathy, left ventricular hypertrophy, and congestive heart failure)

10.9.3 Pathology of nephrosclerosis

- Vascular wall medial thickening, arteriolar hyaline deposits, intimal fibrosis
- Focal glomerular ischemic changes with variable thickening and wrinkling of the basement membranes
- Segmental or global sclerosis, subtotal podocyte foot process effacement
- Tubular atrophy and interstitial fibrosis

10.9.4 Goals of therapy to delay progression of renal failure

- Control blood pressure (achieving target blood pressure is more important to protection of renal function than the selection of particular class of antihypertensive used)
- Reduce albuminuria (when present, ACEI or ARB or perhaps aliskiren is indicated, the role of spironolactone or possibly statins remains to be clarified)
- Low sodium and possibly "Mediterranean" vegetarian diet

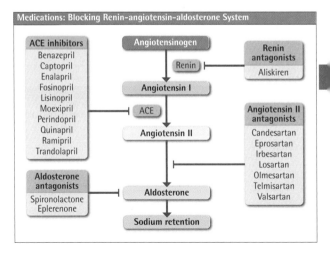

Medications: Blocking Renin-angiotensin-aldosterone System

ACE inhibitors
Benazepril
Captopril
Enalapril
Fosinopril
Lisinopril
Moexipril
Perindopril
Quinapril
Ramipril
Trandolapril

Angiotensinogen

Renin

Renin antagonists
Aliskiren

Angiotensin I

ACE

Angiotensin II

Angiotensin II antagonists
Candesartan
Eprosartan
Irbesartan
Losartan
Olmesartan
Telmisartan
Valsartan

Aldosterone antagonists
Spironolactone
Eplerenone

Aldosterone

Sodium retention

Medications: Affecting Adrenergic Receptors

α 1	Prazosin, terazosin, doxazosin, urapidil
All α receptors	Phentolamine, phenoxybenzamine
α 2	Clonidine, α methyldopa, reserpine, guanfacine
All adrenergic receptors	Labetalol
β1	Atenolol, esmolol, metoprolol, acebutolol*, pindolol*, (*denotes drug has intrinsic beta-agonistic activity)
All β receptors	Propranolol, nadolol, timolol, penbutolol
β 2	Butoxamine (not used in clinical practice)

10.9.5 Classes of calcium channel blockers

Class	Agents	Action & Prevention
Diphenyl-alkylamines	Verapamil HCl	Negative chronotropic actions: Affects sinoatrial and AV nodes to slow conduction and heart rate. Avoid in angina and impaired ventricular function
Benzothiazepines	Diltiazem HCl	Negative chronotropic actions: Affects sinoatrial and AV nodes to slow conduction and heart rate. Avoid in angina and impaired ventricular function
Dihydropyridines	Nifedipine, nicardipine, isradipine, nimodipine, nisoldipine, felodipine, amlodipine besylate	Negative inotropic actions, vasodilators. In systolic dysfunction - avoid nifedipine, but amlodipine and felodipine are acceptable

Class (cont.)	Agents	Action & Prevention
Tetralols	Mibefradil di-hydrochloride	Negatively affects sinoatrial and AV nodes so avoid in AV block or sick sinus syndrome, but not negatively inotropic
Others	Bepridil HCl	Negatively affects sinoatrial and AV nodes so avoid in AV block or sick sinus syndrome and prolongs the QT interval → proarrhythmic

10.9.6 Combinations of calcium channel blockers with beta–blockers

- When combining a CCB with a beta-blocker, a dihydropyridine CCB is desirable as the compensatory tachycardia of the dihydropyridine CCB is opposed by beta-blockade whereas verapamil, diltiazem, or mibefradil added to a beta-blocker is undesirable due to the common side effect of negative chronotropy

10.9.7 Diuretics

Thiazides	Loop diuretics	Potassium sparing	Other
• Chlorothiazide • Chlorthalidone • Hydrochloro-thiazide • Polythiazide • Indapamide • Metolazone	• Bu-metanide • Furose-mide • Torsemide	• Amiloride • Triamterene • Spironolac-tone • Eplerenone	• Carbonic anhydrase inhibitors (acetazol-amide): To induce bicarbonaturia to correct metabolic alkalosis • Osmotic diuretic (manni-tol): Used neurologically for cerebral edema and for some poisonings • Vasopressin receptor antagonists (tolvaptan, conivaptan): To induce a water diuresis for correction of hyponatremia in high ADH states

References and Suggested Reading

Staging, evaluation and treatment of hypertension

The Seventh Report of the Joint National Committee on Prevention, Detection, Evaluation, and Treatment of High Blood Pressure. August, 2004. http://www.nhlbi.nih.gov/guidelines/hypertension/jnc7full.pdf. Accessed October 8, 2012.

Chobanian AV, Bakris GL, Black HR, et al. The Seventh Report of the Joint National Committee on Prevention, Detection, Evaluation, and Treatment of High Blood Pressure: the JNC 7 report. JAMA 2003;289:2560-72.

Sheikh S, Sinha AD, Agarwal R. Home blood pressure monitoring: how good a predictor of long-term risk? Curr Hypertens Rep 2011;13:192-9.

Hodgkinson J, Mant J, Martin U, et al. Relative effectiveness of clinic and home blood pressure monitoring compared with ambulatory blood pressure monitoring in diagnosis of hypertension: systematic review. BMJ 2011;342:d3621.

Minutolo R, Agarwal R, Borrelli S, et al. Prognostic role of ambulatory blood pressure measurement in patients with nondialysis chronic kidney disease. Arch Intern Med. 2011 Jun 27;171(12):1090-8.

Mancia G, De Backer G, Dominiczak A, Cifkova R, et al. 2007 Guidelines for the management of arterial hypertension: The task force for the management of arterial hypertension of the European Society of Hypertension (ESH) and of the European Society of Cardiology (ESC). J Hypertens. 2007;25(6):1105-87.

The ALLHAT Officers and Coordinators for the ALLHAT Collaborative Research Group. Major outcomes in high-risk hypertensive patients randomized to angiotensin-converting enzyme inhibitor or calcium channel blocker vs diuretic: The Antihypertensive and Lipid-Lowering Treatment to Prevent Heart Attack Trial (ALLHAT). JAMA 2002;288:2981-97.

Anand S, Kurella Tamura M. Combining angiotensin receptor blockers with ACE inhibitors in elderly patients. Am J Kidney Dis. 2012; 59(1):11-4.

Shafiq MM, Menon DV, Victor RG. Oral direct renin inhibition: premise, promise, and potential limitations of a new antihypertensive drug. Am J Med 2008; 121:265

Azizi M, Ménard J. Renin inhibitors and cardiovascular and renal protection: an endless quest? Cardiovasc Drugs Ther 2012; Mar 6, PMID: 22392185

Harel Z, Gilbert C, Wald R, et al. The effect of combination treatment with aliskiren and blockers of the renin-angiotensin system on hyperkalaemia and acute kidney injury: systematic review and meta-analysis. BMJ 2012; 344:doi: 10.1136/bmj.e42

Powers BJ, Coeytaux RR, Dolor RJ, et al. Updated report on comparative effectiveness of ACE inhibitors, ARBs, and direct renin inhibitors for patients with essential hypertension: much more data, little new information. J Gen Intern Med. 2012; 27(6):716-29.

Ernst ME, Gordon JA. Diuretic therapy: key aspects in hypertension and renal disease. J Nephrol 2010; 23(5):487-93.

Karadsheh F, Weir MR. Thiazide and thiazide-like diuretics: an opportunity to reduce blood pressure in patients with advanced kidney disease. Curr Hypertens Rep 2012; 14(5):416-20.

Smetana GW. Newer is not always better: all antihypertensive medications do not equally reduce cardiovascular risk. J Gen Intern Med. 2012; 27(6):618-20.

Adams M, Bellone JM, Wright BM, Rutecki GW. Evaluation and pharmacologic approach to patients with resistant hypertension. Postgrad Med 2012; 124(1):74-82.

Acelajado MC, Calhoun DA. Resistant hypertension, secondary hypertension, and hypertensive crises: diagnostic evaluation and treatment. Cardiol Clin 2010; 28(4):639-54.

Kalaitzidis RG, Elisaf MS. The role of statins in chronic kidney disease. Am J Nephrol 2011;34:195-202.

References and Suggested Reading

Young WF. Primary aldosteronism: renaissance of a syndrome. Clin Endocrinol (Oxf) 2007;66(5):607-618.

Heerspink HJL, Holtkamp FA, Parving HH, et al. Moderation of dietary sodium potentiates the renal and cardiovascular protective effects of angiotensin receptor blockers. Kidney Internat 2012; 82(3):330-7.

KDIGO clinical practice guidelines for management of blood pressure in chronic kidney disease. Kidney Int Suppl 2012; 2(5):337-414.

Pacak K. Preoperative management of the pheochromocytoma patient. J Clin Endocrinol Metab. 2007;92(11):4069-4079.

Hypertensive renal disease, renal artery stenosis, and investigational treatments

Udani S, Lazich I, Bakris GL. Epidemiology of hypertensive kidney disease. Nat Rev Nephrol 2010;7:11-21.

Marcantoni C, Fogo AB. A perspective on arterionephrosclerosis: from pathology to potential pathogenesis. J Nephrol 2007;20:518-24.

Hart PD, Bakris GL. Hypertensive nephropathy: prevention and treatment recommendations. Expert Opin Pharmacother 2010;11:2675-86.

Bidani AK, Griffin KA. Pathophysiology of hypertensive renal damage: implications for therapy. Hypertension 2004;44:595-601.

Bomback AS, Muskala P, Bald E, Chwatko G, Nowicki M. Low-dose spironolactone, added to long-term ACE inhibitor therapy, reduces blood pressure and urinary albumin excretion in obese patients with hypertensive target organ damage. Clin Nephrol 2009;72:449-56.

Lao D, Parasher PS, Cho KC, Yeghiazarians Y. Atherosclerotic renal artery stenosis--diagnosis and treatment. Mayo Clin Proc 2011;86:649-57.

Simon JF. Stenting atherosclerotic renal arteries: time to be less aggressive. Cleve Clin J Med 2010;77: 178-89.

Schlaich MP, Sobotka PA, Krum H, et al. Renal sympathetic-nerve ablation for uncontrolled hypertension. N Engl J Med 2009; 361(9):932-4.

Symplicity HTN-1 Investigators. Catheter-based renal sympathetic denervation for resistant hypertension: durability of blood pressure reduction out to 24 months. Hypertension 2011; 57(5):911-7.

Scheffers IJ, Kroon AA, Schmidli J, et al. Novel baroreflex activation therapy in resistant hypertension: results of a European multi-center feasibility study. J Am Coll Cardiol 2010; 56(15):1254-8.

11 Kidney Stones

11.1 Types & Predisposing Causes of Kidney Stones

Kidney Stone Composition Urinary crystal photomicrographs	Percentage of Stones (approx.)	Predisposing Causes
Calcium oxalate (or may be mixed with calcium phosphate)		
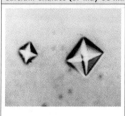	70% (more common in men)	• Hypercalciuria • Hyperuricosuria • Hyperoxaluria • Hypocitraturia • Hypercalcemic states (primary hyperparathyroidism, vitamin D/calcium overdose) • Anatomic kidney abnormalities (eg, medullary sponge kidney) • Low fluid intake and certain diets (increased animal protein, sugar or fructose beverages, or high dose vitamin C intake)
Calcium phosphate		
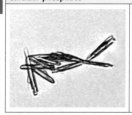	10%	• Hypercalciuria • Type1 RTA • Hypercalcemic states (primary hyperparathyroidism, vitamin D/calcium overdose) • Anatomic kidney abnormalities (eg, medullary sponge kidney)

Kidney Stone Composition Urinary crystal photomicrographs	Percentage of Stones (approx.)	Predisposing Causes
Uric acid		
	10% in USA Up to 40% in hot 'stone belt' areas	• Hyperuricosuria • Chronic diarrheal conditions (uric acid excreted in a decreased volume of highly concentrated acidic urine to compensate for stool losses of $NaHCO_3$)
Struvite or "infection stone" (magnesium ammonium phosphate and calcium carbonate-apatite)		
 	< 5% (more common in women)	Chronic urinary tract infection with a urea-splitting organism (eg, Proteus or Klebsiella)

Kidney Stone Composition Urinary crystal photomicrographs	Percentage of Stones (approx.)	Predisposing Causes
Cystine		
	<1% (more common in children)	Cystinuria
Drugs		
	<1%	• Indinavir • Triamterene • Acyclovir high-dose Rx (urinary crystal shown)

11.2 Presenting Symptoms & Signs

- Flank pain, severe and colicky in nature
- Pain often accompanied by restlessness, nausea and vomiting
- Hematuria, gross or microscopic
- Stone passage: May be felt, but best to strain urine to catch stone

11.3   Detection of Kidney Stones

Noncontrast CT is best (virtually all stones are radioopaque and can usually evaluate obstruction without radiocontrast), US less sensitive but can evaluate obstruction, abdominal x-ray (KUB) can only detect radioopaque larger calcium-containing and some cystine stones, IVP less sensitive than CT and requires radiocontrast

11.4   Initial Workup of Kidney Stone

- History and exam for predisposing risk factors
- Serum electrolytes, calcium, phosphate, creatinine (r/o RTA, hypercalcemia, evaluate renal function)
- Urinalysis to look for hematuria, infection, crystals
- Stone analysis if stone is available
- Radiology: See Detection above, but if medullary sponge kidney is to be detected because there are multiple small stones or nephrocalcinosis, either CT or IVP with radiocontrast will be needed
- Assess daily urine volume output (UO of less than 1 L/day is common and often only Rx for first stone is to increase to 2 L/day)
- Metabolic workup to include 24-h urine studies: Often undertaken after recurrent stone formation or severe first presentation of stone episode

11.5   General Principles of Therapy for Stone Disease

11.5.1   Acute therapy

- Pain relief: NSAIDs, narcotic analgesics
- Intravenous fluid in dehydrated patients, also increases urine flow
- 80% of stones 7mm or less will pass without intervention
- Medications that increase successful stone passage: Alpha-blockers (tamsulosin), calcium channel blockers (nifedipine most commonly)

11.5.2   Indications for hospitalization/interventional procedure

- Intractable pain and vomiting
- Severe urinary tract infection or sepsis
- Complete ureteral obstruction for >3 days
- Partial obstruction of a solitary kidney
- Obstruction or infection may indicate need for temporary ureteral stent placement or nephrostomy

11.5.3   Urologic interventions

- Extracorporeal shock wave lithotripsy (ESWL) has better success with smaller stones
- Ureteroscopic lithotripsy (useful for ureteral stones)
- Percutaneous nephrolithotomy (successful on larger stones but with increased complication rate than lithotripsy, equal success to open surgical procedures)
- Laparoscopic or open surgical stone removal

11.5.4 General stone management

- Specific stone therapy as noted below when stone composition is known
- Fluid intake to increase urine output to >2 L/day
- Dietary considerations
  - Reduce fructose and sugar containing beverage consumption which may increase calcium stone occurrence
  - Replace sweet and dairy fluids with coffee, tea and water
  - Reduce high intake of vitamin D and calcium supplementation but maintain normal calcium diet
  - Reduce intake of animal protein

11.5.5 Follow-up

- Reassess effects of specific therapy when indicated with urinary and plasma chemistries in 2 months and yearly
- Consider radiologic assessment for new stone formation at 1 year
- Whenever recurrent stone disease is uncomplicated by infection, obstruction, or underlying disorders, the major risks for patients are the occurrence of painful episodes and the possibility of requiring urologic interventions for stone passage. In general, renal function has been thought to be well preserved, but recent data suggests that those with one or more kidney stones have about double the risk of developing CKD or ESRD, with the added hazard appearing to be greater in women than in men.

11.6 Predisposing Causes of Stone Formation

Hypercalciuria or Idiopathic Hypercalciuria
Defining the Defect
Urinary calcium: • In men: >300 mg/d ,   • In women >250 mg/d, or   • >4 mg/Kg/d in children and small adults
Mechanisms Involved
• **Absorptive :** Increased GI absorption of calcium - can be assessed by urinary calcium to creatinine ratio of >0.2 mg/mg after an oral calcium load   • **Resorptive:** Increased bone resorption - may have elevated PTH without hypercalcemia   • **Renal "leak":** Decrease in renal tubular calcium reabsorption - can be assessed by fasting urinary calcium >0.11 mg/100 ml/min of CrCl   • **Hypophosphatemic:** Renal phosphate wasting may stimulate increased 1,25-dihydroxy-vitamin D, enhancing GI absorption of calcium

Hypercalciuria or Idiopathic Hypercalciuria (cont.)

Treatment of Specific Causes of Recurrent Stones

Bone density studies of hypercalciuric patients have generally shown decreased bone density in all of the 4 mechanistic categories listed above, making evaluation of mechanism clinically unnecessary, with treatment as follows:

• Reduce dietary Na to <2 g/day to increase renal tubular reabsorption of calcium
• Maintain a normal, rather than a low, calcium diet to bind dietary oxalates and avoid osteopenia but avoid added calcium and vitamin D products
• Thiazide diuretics (eg, hydrochlorothiazide, 25-50 mg twice a day) decreases urinary calcium excretion by about 50% with a demonstrated reduction in stone incidence
• Avoid hypokalemia which reduces urinary citrate - potassium citrate may be used to prevent thiazide-induced hypocitraturia
• Amiloride can be used with a thiazide instead of potassium citrate to reduce urinary excretion of both potassium and calcium
• An alternative therapy, neutral sodium phosphate (500 mg four times a day) corrects the low serum phosphate in the hypophosphatemic form of hypercalciuria which may decrease calcium excretion. It also increases urinary pyrophosphate excretion to solubilize calcium, but has not been shown to decrease stone occurrence

Hypocitraturia

Defining the Defect

• Urinary citrate <320 mEq/d

Mechanisms Involved

• Idiopathic or associated with RTA, cystic fibrosis, chronic metabolic acidosis (diarrhea, carbonic anhydrase inhibitors)

Treatment of Specific Causes of Recurrent Stones

• Potassium citrate has been demonstrated to decrease stone occurrence (10-20 mEq); 3 times a day for urinary citrate <320 mEq/d, 20 mEq 3-4 times a day for urinary citrate <150 mEq/d)

Hyperuricosuria (may be associated with either uric acid or calcium oxalate stones)

Defining the Defect

• Urinary uric acid >750-800 mg/d
Note: Uric acid stones can occur with normal excretion of uric acid due to low urine pH in chronic diarrheal states.

Mechanisms Involved

• Overproduction of uric acid may occur with or without gout, certain enzyme defects, high purine intake, myeloproliferative and hemolytic disorders, cytotoxic drugs, and alcoholism

Treatment of Specific Causes of Recurrent Stones

• For hyperuricosuria, allopurinol has been shown to decrease both uric acid and calcium oxalate stone occurrence
• For uric acid stones with normal uric acid excretion or with intolerance to allopurinol or febuxostat, alkalinize the urine to pH >6.5 to increase urate solubility ($NaHCO_3$ or sodium or potassium citrate, 1-3 mEq/Kg/day, usually given in 4 doses). Urinary alkalinization is highly effective and can dissolve uric acid stones, if adherence is maintained.
• Avoid purine-rich foods

Cystinuria

Defining the Defect

• Urinary cystine >400 mg/d or cystine crystals in urinary sediment
• Cystine stone formation

Mechanisms Involved

• Several genetic defects in cystine and dibasic amino acid transport decreasing renal tubular cystine reabsorption

Treatment of Specific Causes of Recurrent Stones

• Dietary protein and sodium restriction decreases urinary cystine
• Alkalinization of urine to pH >7.0-7.5 with potassium citrate
• Bedtime dose of acetazolamide or potassium citrate to maintain alkaline urine at night
• Fluid intake to very high urine output >3-4 L/d
If those measures fail:
• Thiol drug treatment with penicillamine or tiopronin (or perhaps captopril) to decrease cystine by forming cysteine-drug disulfide bonds has been shown to decrease cystine stone occurrence

Hyperoxaluria

Defining the Defect

Urinary oxalate >45 mg/d

Mechanisms Involved

- Primary hyperoxaluria (3 types of genetic defects - rare but overproduction may be as much as >>100 mg/d)
- May be associated with idiopathic hypercalciuria
- Secondary: Intestinal hyperabsorption in malabsorption syndromes, post-bypass surgery, inflammatory bowel disease, pancreatic insufficiency, and cystic fibrosis
- High-dose vitamin C intake increases endogenous oxalate production

Treatment of Specific Causes of Recurrent Stones

- Low-oxalate diet (restrict dietary intake of spinach and other leafy vegetables, cranberries, tea, cocoa and nuts)
- Avoid high-dose vitamin C

To decrease intestinal absorption of oxalate:
- Low-fat diet helps reduce free oxalate in the intestine
- Calcium carbonate or citrate, 1 to 4 g/d with meals, binds oxalate in the intestine with a greater proportional decrease in urinary oxalate than increase in urinary calcium
- Cholestyramine, an oxalate-binding resin, at a dose of 8 to 16 g/d may help
- Restoration of small bowel continuity, if possible (if prior bypass surgery)

For primary hyperoxaluria:
- Pyridoxine at high dose (100 - 800 mg/d) for hereditary deficiency type 1
- Neutral sodium phosphate and potassium citrate as above may help decrease urinary supersaturation of calcium oxalate
- Segmental liver transplant, to correct the enzyme defect, combined with a kidney transplant for renal failure, has been successfully utilized in patients with hereditary hyperoxaluria

Struvite Crystalluria (magnesium ammonium phosphate)
Defining the Defect
• Chronic urinary infection with a urea-splitting organism, urine pH > 7.0, struvite stone or staghorn
Mechanisms Involved
• Urease producing bacteria break down urea to ammonia leading to alkaline urine and struvite crystallization with calcium carbonate and phosphate
Treatment of Specific Causes of Recurrent Stones
• Eradication of infection, if possible, with long-term antimicrobial therapy
• Urease inhibitor therapy (acetohydroxamic acid decreases stone formation but often causes side effects)
• Removal of stones with lithotripsy, percutaneous nephrolithotomy, or open surgery
• Evaluate for an underlying additional stone-forming disorder, eg, hypercalciuria

References and Suggested Reading

Sakhaee K, Maalouf NM, Sinnott B. Clinical review. Kidney stones: pathogenesis, diagnosis, and management. J Clin Endocrinol Metab 2012; 97(6):1847-60.

Fink HA, Wilt TJ, Eidman KE, et al. Medical management to prevent recurrent nephrolithiasis in adults: A systematiic review for an American College of Physicians clinical guideline. Ann Intern Med 2013; 158(7):535-543.

Worcester EM, Coe FL. Clinical practice: Calcium kidney stones. N Engl J Med 2010; 363(10):954-63.

Schade GR, Faerber GJ. Urinary tract stones. Prim Care 2010; 37(3):565-81, ix.

Hoppe B, Kemper MJ. Diagnostic examination of the child with urolithiasis or nephrocalcinosis. Pediatr Nephrol 2010; 25(3):403-13.

Mandeville JA, Gnessin E Lingeman JE. Imaging evaluation in the patient with renal stone disease. Semin Nephrol 2011; 31(3):254-8.

Johri N, Cooper B, Robertson W, et al. An update and practical guide to renal stone management. Nephron Clin Pract 2010; 116(3):c159-71.

Sakhaee K. Recent advances in the pathophysiology of nephrolithiasis. Kidney Int 2009; 75(6):585-95.

Katabathina VS, Kota G, Dasyam AK, et al. Adult renal cystic disease: a genetic, biological, and developmental primer. Radiographics 2010; 30(6):1509-23

Srisubat A, Potisat S, Lojanapiwat B, et al. Extracorporeal shock wave lithotripsy (ESWL) versus percutaneous nephrolithotomy (PCNL) or retrograde intrarenal surgery (RIRS) for kidney stones. Cochrane Database Syst Rev (2009)(4): CD007044.

Alexander RT, Hemmelgarn BR, Wiebe N, et al for the Alberta Kidney Disease Network. Kidney stones and kidney function loss: a cohort study. BMJ 2012;345:e5287 doi: 10.1136/bmj.e5287

Moe OW, Pearle MS, Sakhaee K. Pharmacotherapy of urolithiasis: evidence from clinical trials. Kidney Int 2011; 79(4):385-92.

Reilly RF, Peixoto AJ, Desir GV. The evidence-based use of thiazide diuretics in hypertension and nephrolithiasis. Clin J Am Soc Nephrol 2010; 5(10):1893-903.

El-Zoghby ZM, Lieske JC, Foley RN, et al. Urolithiasis and the risk of ESRD. Clin J Am Soc Nephrol 2012; 7(9):1409-15.

Coe FL, Evan A, Worcester E. Pathophysiology-based treatment of idiopathic calcium kidney stones. Clin J Am Soc Nephrol. 2011 Aug 6(8):2083-92

Goldfarb DS. A woman with recurrent calcium phosphate kidney stones. Clin J Am Soc Nephrol 2012 Jul 7(7):1172-78.

Thomas LDK, Elinder CG, Tiselius HG, et al. Ascorbic Acid Supplements and Kidney Stone Incidence Among Men: A Prospective Study. JAMA Intern Med 2013; 1-2. doi:10.1001/jamainternmed.2013.2296.

Prié D, Friedlander G. Genetic disorders of renal phosphate transport. N Engl J Med 2010; 362(25): 2399-409.

Goldfarb DS. Potential pharmacologic treatments for cystinuria and for calcium stones associated with hyperuricosuria. Clin J Am Soc Nephrol 2011; 6(8):2093-7.

12   Acute Kidney Injury/Acute Renal Failure

12.1   Definition of AKI

- Increase in SCr by ≥0.3 mg/dl within 48 hours; or
- Increase in SCr to ≥1.5 times baseline, which is known or presumed to have occurred within the prior 7 days; or
- Urine volume <0.5 ml/Kg/h for 6 hours.

12.2   Staging of AKI

The following definition of stages of AKI was proposed by KDIGO group as a single definition to replace similar staging systems by RIFLE and AKIN. Remember that formulae designed for calculating eGFR or creatinine clearance from serum creatinine levels must not be used in patients with AKI or any case in which the serum level is unstable.

Stage	Serum Creatinine	Urine Output
1	1.5-1.9 times baseline OR ≥0.3 mg/dl (≥26.5 mmol/l) increase	<0.5 ml/Kg/h for 6-12 hours
2	2.0-2.9 times baseline	<0.5 ml/Kg/h for ≥12 hours
3	3.0 times baseline OR Increase in serum creatinine to ≥4.0 mg/dl OR Initiation of renal replacement therapy OR In patients <18 years, decrease in eGFR to <35 ml/min per 1.73 m^2	<0.3 ml/Kg/h for ≥24 hours OR Anuria for ≥12 hours

KDIGO Clinical Practice Guideline for Acute Kidney Injury

12.3 KDIGO Clinical Practice Guideline for Acute Kidney Injury (AKI)

Using the stages of AKI severity listed above, the KDIGO guidelines suggest general evaluation and management strategies as shown in the following algorithms:

Stage-based Management of AKI

	AKI Stage		
High Risk	**1**	**2**	**3**
Discontinue all nephrotoxic agent when possible			
Ensure volume status and perfusion pressure			
Consider functional hemodynamic monitoring			
Monitor serum creatinine and urine output			
Avoid hyperglycemia			
Consider alternatives to radiocontrast procedures			
	Non-invasive diagnostic workup		
	Consider invasive diagnostic workup		
		Check for changes in drug dosing	
		Consider Renal Replacement Theraphy	
		Consider ICU admission	
			Avoid subclavian catheters if possible

Shading of boxes indicates priority of action — solid shading indicates actions that are equally appropriate at all stages whereas graded shading indicates increasing priority as intensity increases. AKI, acute kidney injury; ICU, intensive-care unit.

KDIGO Clinical Practice Guideline for Acute Kidney Injury

Evaluation of AKI According to the Stage and Cause

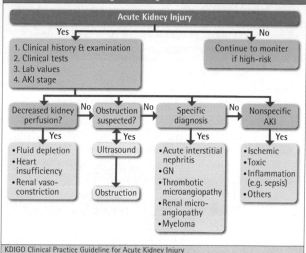

KDIGO Clinical Practice Guideline for Acute Kidney Injury

12.4   Incidence & Mortality Rate of AKI

It appears that the incidence of AKI in hospitalized patients has been rising over the past two decades. In one study of a representative nationwide sample of over 5 million inpatients discharged with ARF or ARF that required dialysis (ARF-D) between 1988 and 2002, the incidence of ARF increased from 61 to 288 per 100,000 population, and ARF-D increased from 4 to 27 per 100,000 population. However, over the same 15 years, the mortality rate of ARF declined from 40.4% to 20.3% and that of ARF-D declined from 41.3% to 28.1%, as shown on the graphs below. The increase of almost 7-fold of inpatients requiring dialysis suggests that the increased incidence of ARF is not explained by a change of diagnostic criteria over time, but a real rise of kidney injuries, likely caused by many of the multiple factors described in this chapter in the setting of better resuscitative medical management and increased use of nephrotoxic agents.

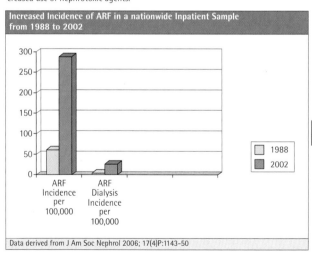

Increased Incidence of ARF in a nationwide Inpatient Sample from 1988 to 2002

Data derived from J Am Soc Nephrol 2006; 17(4)P:1143-50

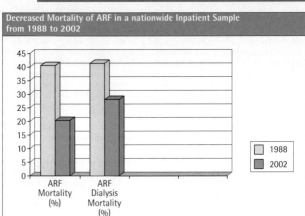

Decreased Mortality of ARF in a nationwide Inpatient Sample from 1988 to 2002

Data derived from J Am Soc Nephrol 2006; 17(4)P:1143-50

This increase in the incidence of AKI requiring dialysis has continued up to 2009 as shown in the next figure. The rise was seen in all age groups, races, and both sexes, though older individuals, blacks and males were at greatest risk.

Population Incidence of Dialysis-requiring AKI in United States from 2000 to 2009 (absolute count & incidence rate per million person-years)

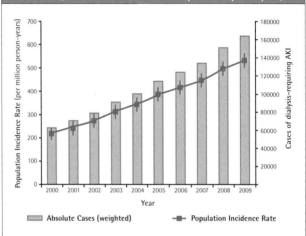

Legend: Absolute Cases (weighted) — Population Incidence Rate

Hsu RK, McCulloch CE, Dudley RA, et al. Temporal changes in incidence of dialysis-requiring AKI. J Am Soc Nephrol 2013; 24(1): 37–42.

Moreover, it has been recognized that even small increments in the serum creatinine, as little as a ≥ 0.3-0.5 mg/dL rise, in general hospital patients or after cardiac surgery are associated with several fold increases in the mortality rate, and this increase may persist for up to 10 years following acute myocardial infarction.

12.5   Initial Diagnostic Approach to AKI

Initial step in the diagnostic approach to patient with kidney insufficiency is to determine if the injury is acute or chronic.

Source of Information	Acute	Chronic
Medical History	Abrupt ↑ in S_{Cr} over days	Slow increase in S_{Cr} over weeks to months
Symptoms	Recent onset of symptoms, eg, fever, flank pain, decreased or discolored urine	No symptoms or slow onset of fatigue, anorexia, weakness, nausea, and/or pruritus
Labs	Further ↑ in S_{Cr} after initial evaluation	Relatively stable S_{Cr}
Anemia	Less typical or secondary to other than renal causes	More typical although not very specific
Ultrasound	Normal or enlarged size kidneys	Small kidneys with increased echogenicity, although may be of normal size, particularly with diabetes, amyloidosis, or polycystic kidney disease

12.6 Diagnostic Steps to Establish the Cause of AKI

Acute Kidney Injury: Causes

Diagnostic steps

- History, prior medical records, physical exam
- Urine output measurement: Oliguria <400 ml/24h or anuria <100 ml/24h (no urine or absolute anuria is diagnostically significant and usually caused by shock, complete urinary tract obstruction, bilateral renovascular occlusion, or HUS/TTP with renal cortical necrosis)
- Foley catheter to measure output if oligo-anuric
- Urinalysis
- Urinary indices (see below)
- Ultrasound of urinary tract ± Doppler
- Rate of rise in S_{Cr} over time (ie, 0.4–2.0 mg/dl per day rise in ATN; less and often variable in prerenal azotemia)

- Evaluation of intravascular volume and cardiac output
- Additional blood tests (Hep B, Hep C, lupus, myeloma w/u)
- Renal vascular studies (radioisotope scan, MRA, angiography)
- Gallium scan – positive with strong uptake in AIN, negative in ATN
- Therapeutic trials as indicated: volume expansion, inotropic agents, diuretic trial (may increase UO but doesn't increase GFR), relief of ureteral obstruction (ie, SCr improves within 24–72 h with improved renal perfusion in prerenal azotemia, but does not in ATN)

- Kidney biopsy
- Empiric therapy for suspected disease, e.g., corticosteroids for AIN

12.7 Diagnostic Algorithm for AKI

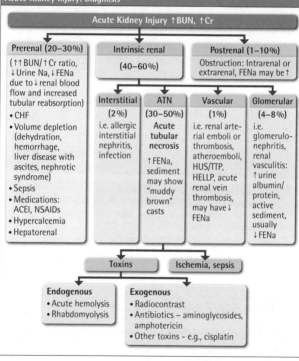

Acute Kidney Injury: Diagnosis

Acute Kidney Injury ↑BUN, ↑Cr

Prenal (20–30%)

(↑↑BUN/↑Cr ratio, ↓Urine Na, ↓FENa due to ↓renal blood flow and increased tubular reabsorption)
- CHF
- Volume depletion (dehydration, hemorrhage, liver disease with ascites, nephrotic syndrome)
- Sepsis
- Medications: ACEI, NSAIDs
- Hypercalcemia
- Hepatorenal

Intrinsic renal (40–60%)

Interstitial (2%)
i.e. allergic interstitial nephritis, infection

ATN (30–50%)
Acute tubular necrosis
↑FENa, sediment may show "muddy brown" casts

Vascular (1%)
i.e. renal arterial emboli or thrombosis, atheroemboli, HUS/TTP, HELLP, acute renal vein thrombosis, may have ↓FENa

Glomerular (4–8%)
i.e. glomerulonephritis, renal vasculitis: ↑urine albumin/protein, active sediment, usually ↓FENa

Postrenal (1–10%)
Obstruction: Intrarenal or extrarenal, FENa may be ↑

Toxins

Ischemia, sepsis

Endogenous
- Acute hemolysis
- Rhabdomyolysis

Exogenous
- Radiocontrast
- Antibiotics – aminoglycosides, amphotericin
- Other toxins – e.g., cisplatin

12.8 Red Flags

While most cases of AKI are due to either prerenal conditions or ATN, one should be able to identify "red flags" for other potential etiologies of AKI. In addition, do not miss urinary obstruction - kidney ultrasound should be done in most of AKI cases.

Signs and Symptoms	Potential Etiology
Proteinuria and hematuria	Glomerulonephritis, AIN
Heavy proteinuria (> 3 g/d)	Glomerulonephritis, renal vein thrombosis
Thrombocytopenia	HUS/TTP, HELLP, DIC
Lung infiltrates/nodules, hemoptysis, ARF	Pulmonary renal syndromes - see below
Purpura (palpable purpura)	HSP, other forms of vasculitis, cryoglobulinemia
Skin rash	AIN, SLE
Very high blood pressure	Scleroderma crisis, malignant hypertension
Joint pain	SLE, rheumatoid arthritis, HSP

12.9 Urinary Indices in Acute Renal Failure (ARF)

Urinary indices and other signs to differentiate between prerenal azotemia and ATN (FE = fractional excretion)

Lab Test	Prerenal Azotemia	ATN
Urine to Plasma Cr ratio	>40	<20
BUN/Cr ratio	>20	<10-15
$U_{Urea\ nitrogen}$/BUN	>8	<3
UNa (mEq/l)	<20	>40
FENa (%)	<1	>2
FE uric acid (%) - useful when on loop diuretics	<7	>15
Urinalysis	Hyaline casts or negative sediment	Abnormal: Muddy brown granular & renal tubular epithelial cell casts, free renal tubular epithelial cells
Specific gravity	>1.020	~1.010
U_{osm} (mOsm/kg H2O)	>500	<350-450

None of the above criteria of prerenal disease may be present in patients with underlying chronic renal disease since their ability to concentrate the urine might be impaired by the CKD.

FENa

FENa is probably the urinary index most commonly used in the work-up of AKI

$$FE_{Na} = \frac{Na^+ \text{ excreted}}{Na^+ \text{ filtered}} = \frac{(U_{Na} \times S_{Cr} \times 100)}{(S_{Na} \times U_{Cr})}$$

When FeNa might not be helpful (ie, poor specificity)	
↑ FeNa in prerenal ARF or other non-ATN azotemia	↓ FeNa in ATN or other non-pre-renal azotemia
• Diuretics • Osmotic agents: Radiocontrast, glucose, urea • Adrenal insufficiency • Underlying chronic renal insufficiency • Underlying interstitial disease • Acute volume expansion with ↑ Na excretion • Obstructive uropathy	• Underlying chronic prerenal disease (hepato-renal syndrome, CHF) • Early in the course of ATN secondary to sepsis, ischemia ("intermediate" syndrome with features of both ATN and prerenal failure) radiocontrast, hemolysis, rhabdomyolysis • AIN, acute GN, vasculitis • Renal artery occlusion

BUN/Cr

Another index is the BUN/Cr ratio. Normally it is ranging about 10–20. However in certain conditions BUN and Cr levels might change disproportionately.

Disproportional BUN/Cr Ratio	
↑ BUN/Cr	↓ BUN/Cr
• Prerenal failure • GI bleeding • Catabolic states • Antianabolic agents • Postrenal obstruction • ↓Cr with ↓ muscle mass in elderly or paralyzed patient • Steroids and tetracycline	• Hepatic insufficiency • Rhabdomyolysis • Malnutrition

12.10 Acute Tubular Necrosis (ATN)

Causes of ATN	
Ischemic	Toxicity
• Sepsis • Hypovolemia (GI, renal or skin losses, bleeding), hypotension • Decreased renal plasma flow in edematous states (CHF, cirrhosis, hepatorenal syndrome, nephrotic syndrome) • Medications (ACEI, calcineurin inhibitors, NSAIDs, amphotericin, radiocontrast) • Renal vascular disease (renal artery thrombosis, stenosis, or embolization; atheroemboli, HUS, other forms of vasculitis or small vessel injury including transplant rejection, sickle cell anemia, preeclampsia, malignant HTN)	• Gentamicin, vancomycin, amphotericin, other drugs (see 12.12 below →195) • Radiocontrast • Hemoglobin (hemolysis) • Myoglobin (rhabdomyolysis) • Other toxins (eg, heavy metals, ethylene glycol)

12.11 Contrast-induced Nephropathy (CIN)

12.11.1 Definition

Increase in the serum creatinine concentration of 0.5 mg/dL or a 25% increase from baseline within 3 days after the administration of contrast media in the absence of an alternative cause.

12.11.2 Natural history

• SCr concentration increases within 24 to 48 hours of exposure and peaks at 3 to 5 days
• Impaired renal function resolves, usually within 7 -10 days
• Renal impairment of later onset and prolonged duration: Look for other causes

12.11.3 Incidence

• Approx 0.5% of patients with normal kidney function
• 10-40% of patients with preexisting renal insufficiency with arteriography

12.11.4 Pathophysiology of radiocontrast nephropathy

- Compromised renal blood flow which results in medullary ischemia
- Alterations in the metabolism of nitric oxide (NO), adenosine, angiotensin II, and prostaglandins
- Contrast induces osmotic diuresis, and active transport increases renal metabolic activity and oxygen consumption.
- Contrast media stimulates a rapid influx of extracellular calcium leading to prolonged constriction of renal vasculature
- Contrast generates reactive oxygen species, which may also reduce the regional blood flow.
- Contrast can also have direct toxic renal tubular effects.
- High osmolarity results in reduction of renal blood flow.

12.11.5 Risk factors

- Diminished baseline renal function (exponential increase in risk of CIN with rising creatinine)
- Peripheral vascular disease
- Diabetes
- CHF
- Cardiogenic shock
- Volume depletion
- Chronic liver disease
- Volume of contrast agent
- Potentially nephrotoxic drugs (eg, NSAIDs)
- Proteinuria, especially myeloma proteins
- HTN

12.11.6 Prevention

- Limit the dose of contrast
- Use alternative imaging techniques whenever possible
- Volume expansion with either isotonic sodium chloride or sodium bicarbonate solutions
- Pretreatment with n-acetylcysteine (NAC) - conflicting data
- Use of iso-osmolar contrast

12.12 AKI Induced by Medications

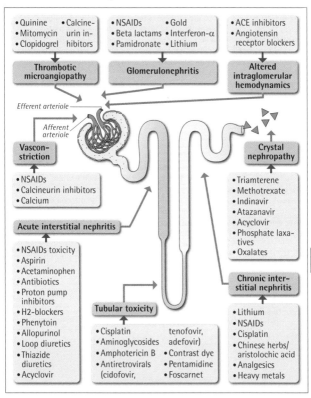

Thrombotic microangiopathy
• Quinine
• Mitomycin
• Clopidogrel
• Calcineurin inhibitors

Glomerulonephritis
• NSAIDs
• Beta lactams
• Pamidronate
• Gold
• Interferon-α
• Lithium

Altered intraglomerular hemodynamics
• ACE inhibitors
• Angiotensin receptor blockers

Efferent arteriole
Afferent arteriole

Vasoconstriction
• NSAIDs
• Calcineurin inhibitors
• Calcium

Crystal nephropathy
• Triamterene
• Methotrexate
• Indinavir
• Atazanavir
• Acyclovir
• Phosphate laxatives
• Oxalates

Acute interstitial nephritis
• NSAIDs toxicity
• Aspirin
• Acetaminophen
• Antibiotics
• Proton pump inhibitors
• H2-blockers
• Phenytoin
• Allopurinol
• Loop diuretics
• Thiazide diuretics
• Acyclovir

Tubular toxicity
• Cisplatin
• Aminoglycosides
• Amphotericin B
• Antiretrovirals (cidofovir, tenofovir, adefovir)
• Contrast dye
• Pentamidine
• Foscarnet

Chronic interstitial nephritis
• Lithium
• NSAIDs
• Cisplatin
• Chinese herbs/ aristolochic acid
• Analgesics
• Heavy metals

12.13 Biomarkers

Numerous biomarkers potentially useful in the diagnosis of ATN have been proposed over the last decade. Clinical use of these biomarkers to this day is limited to research; as the clinical implementation of these diagnostics remains controversial. The most promising biomarkers are summarized in the following table. Most are normally expressed in the proximal tubule, some also by the distal tubule (except for cystatin C - expressed by all nucleated cells), and are measured by ELISA (except for NAG).

Biomarker	Function
Urine/serum neutrophil gelatinase-associated lipocalin (NGAL)	Growth differentiation factor, also participates in iron trafficking, upregulated in ischemic injury and released into urine
Urine kidney injury molecule-1 (KIM-1)	Membrane glycoprotein, shed into urine during acute injury, production increased in response to injury
Urine/serum IL-18	Immunomodulation, inflammation, upregulated in ischemic injury and released into urine
Urine/serum cystatin C	Protein produced by nucleated cells, cysteine protease inhibitor, during injury filtration decreased and proximal tubule metabolism decreases
Urine liver fatty-acid binding protein (L-FABP)	Fatty acid trafficking protein, which translocates from cytosol to tubular lumen during ischemic injury
Plasma IL-6	Immunomodulation, inflammation, the production increased and clearance decreased in association with AKI
Urine alpha glutathione S-transferase (GST)	Cytosolic enzymes released during injury
Urine N-acetyl-beta-glucosaminidase (NAG)	Lysosomal enzyme (glucosidase) expressed in proximal tubules

12.14 Acute Kidney Injury Due to Glomerular Disease

Acute Glomerulonephritis Causing AKI	
Primary GN	**Secondary disease**
• IgA nephropathy • Membranoproliferative nephritis • Postinfectious GN • Collapsing glomerulopathy	• Cryoglobulinemia • Goodpasture's syndrome • Lupus nephritis • Henoch-Schönlein purpura (HSP) • Vasculitis (eg, granulomatosis with polyangiitis (formerly Wegener's), ANCA vasculitis, polyarteritis nodosa)

12.15 Pulmonary–Renal Vasculitic Syndromes

Pulmonary renal syndromes are a subset of diseases causing acute glomerulonephritis and diffuse alveolar hemorrhage. The majority of cases are associated with positive ANCA levels.

• Microscopic polyangiitis, often associated with p-ANCA positivity
• Granulomatosis with polyangiitis (Wegener's), often associated with c-ANCA positivity
• Churg-Strauss syndrome
• Systemic lupus erythematosus with lung involvement
• Goodpasture's syndrome, associated with an anti-GBM antibody
• Behcet's disease
• Rheumatoid vasculitis

12.16 Acute Interstitial Nephritis (AIN)

(See Chap 8.1 →125)

12.16.1 Causes of acute interstitial nephritis

• Infection
  - Bacterial (Corynebacterium diphtheriae, Legionella, staphylococci, streptococci, yersinia)
  - Viral (CMV, EBV, hantavirus, HIV, HSV, hepatitis C, mumps, BK)
  - Other (Leptospira, mycobacterium, mycoplasma, rickettsia, syphilis, toxoplasmosis)
• Immune diseases (SLE, sarcoid, Sjögren syndrome, vasculitis, lymphoproliferative disorders)
• Acute rejection of kidney transplant
• Medications
  - Antivirals
  - Antibiotics (PCN, cephalosporins, rifampin, ciprofloxacin)
  - Sulfa-based drugs (TMP/SMZ, HCTZ, furosemide)
  - Proton pump inhibitors (the most common cause of acute interstitial nephritis)
  - NSAIDs, 5-ASA, others

12.16.2 Diagnosis of AIN

- Light proteinuria (<2 g/day), WBCs in urinary sediment
- Eosinophiluria and/or eosinophilia
- Gallium scan positivity of kidneys
- Kidney biopsy

12.16.3 Treatment of the AIN

- Removing drug responsible for AIN
- Brief course of corticosteroids (as described in Chap 8.1)

12.17 Management of AKI

Treatment of AKI
• First look for reversible causative factors, eg, infection, obstruction, nephrotoxins, circulatory failure, hypercalcemia, etc.
• Supportive care with careful fluid balance and electrolyte balance
• Pharmacologic manipulations (loop diuretics may increase urine output, dopamine for low cardiac output only, most drug trials ineffective)
• Phosphate binders for hyperphosphatemia ($CaCO_3$ if serum Ca is low, aluminum hydroxide or carbonate can be used for acute management without aluminum toxicity in short courses of < 1 month))
• Renal replacement therapy (RRT)

Indications for RRT in ARF
• Symptoms or signs of the uremic syndrome (pericarditis, neuropathy, encephalopathy, seizures, coagulopathy, enteropathy with GI symptoms)
• Refractory hypervolemia
• Severe uncontrolled electrolyte abnormalities (hyperkalemia)
• Severe uncontrolled acid-base disorder (eg, metabolic acidosis)
• Early initiation of dialysis in critically ill patients might be beneficial for survival
• Probability of death is unchanged by intensive vs adequate renal replacement therapy

Potential negative effect of dialysis in ARF
• Decreased urine output caused by removal of volume and urea by dialysis
• Repeated episodes of hypotension (less common with PD & CVVH)
• Complement activation (less severe with biocompatible dialysis membranes)

Nutritional considerations in patients with AKI
• Energy requirements: 35 kcal/Kg/day
• Protein requirements: 1.2 g protein /Kg/day but > 1.25 g/Kg/day not beneficial and will increase rate of BUN rise
• Other nutrients: Ratio between glucose and lipids 70/30 to provide calories
• Usually low Na, low K, low phosphate diet is desirable to control fluid retention, hyperkalemia and hyperphosphatemia

References and Suggested Reading

ARF/AKI definition, staging, incidence and mortality

The 2011 Kidney Disease: Improving Global Outcomes (KDIGO) Clinical Practice Guideline for Acute Kidney Injury (AKI). Kidney International 2012;2, suppl.1:1–138.

Mehta RL, Kellum JA, Shah SV, et al. Acute Kidney Injury Network: report of an initiative to improve outcomes in acute kidney injury. Crit Care 2007;11:R31.

Bellomo R, Ronco C, Kellum JA, Mehta RL, Palevsky P. Acute renal failure - definition, outcome measures, animal models, fluid therapy and information technology needs: the Second International Consensus Conference of the Acute Dialysis Quality Initiative (ADQI) Group. Crit Care 2004;8:R204-12.

Waikar SS, Curhan GC, Wald R et al. Declining mortality in patients with acute renal failure, 1988 to 2002. J Am Soc Nephrol 2006; 17(4):1143-50.

Hsu RK, McCulloch CE, Dudley RA, et al. Temporal changes in incidence of dialysis-requiring AKI. J Am Soc Nephrol 2013; 24(1): 37–42.

Chertow GM, Burdick E, Honour M, et al. Acute kidney injury, mortality, length of stay, and costs in hospitalized patients. J Am Soc Nephrol 2005; 16(11):3365-70.

Lassnigg A, Schmidlin D, Mouhieddine M, et al. Minimal changes of serum creatinine predict prognosis in patients after cardiothoracic surgery: a prospective cohort study. J Am Soc Nephrol 2004; 15(6):1597-605.

Parikh CR, Coca SG, Wang Y, et al. Long-term prognosis of acute kidney injury after acute myocardial infarction. Arch Intern Med 2008; 168(9):987-95.

Ischemic and nephrotoxic ATN

Bonventre JV, Yang L. Cellular pathophysiology of ischemic acute kidney injury. J Clin Invest 2011;121:4210-21.

Ho KM, Power BM. Benefits and risks of furosemide in acute kidney injury. Anaesthesia (2010 Mar) 65(3):283-93.

Nigwekar SU, Waikar SS. Diuretics in acute kidney injury. Semin Nephrol 2011; 31(6):523-34.

Naughton CA. Drug-induced nephrotoxicity. Am Fam Physician 2008;78:743-50.

Gupta A, Biyani M, Khaira A. Vancomycin nephrotoxicity: myths and facts. Neth J Med 2011;69:379-83.

Weisbord SD, Palevsky PM. Contrast-induced acute kidney injury: short- and long-term implications. Semin Nephrol 2011;31:300-9.

Seeliger E, Sendeski M, Rihal CS, Persson PB. Contrast-induced kidney injury: mechanisms, risk factors, and prevention. Eur Heart J 2012; 33(16):2007-15.

Mosca L, Grundy SM, Judelson D, et al. AHA/ACC scientific statement: consensus panel statement. Guide to preventive cardiology for women. American Heart Association/American College of Cardiology. J Am Coll Cardiol 1999;33:1751-5.

Morcos SK. Prevention of contrast media nephrotoxicity--the story so far. Clin Radiol 2004;59:381-9.

Freeman RV, O'Donnell M, Share D, et al. Nephropathy requiring dialysis after percutaneous coronary intervention and the critical role of an adjusted contrast dose. Am J Cardiol 2002;90:1068-73.

Pulmonary renal syndromes

Jara LJ, Vera-Lastra O, Calleja MC. Pulmonary-renal vasculitic disorders: differential diagnosis and management. Curr Rheumatol Rep 2003;5:107-15.

References and Suggested Reading (cont.)

Acute interstitial nephritis

Kodner CM, Kudrimoti A. Diagnosis and management of acute interstitial nephritis. Am Fam Physician 2003;67:2527-34.

Rossert J. Drug-induced acute interstitial nephritis. Kidney Int 2001;60:804-17.

Renal replacement therapy for ARF/AKI

Karvellas CJ, Farhat MR, Sajjad I, et al. A comparison of early versus late initiation of renal replacement therapy in critically ill patients with acute kidney injury: a systematic review and meta-analysis. Crit Care 2011;15:R72.

Palevsky PM, Zhang JH, O'Connor TZ, et al. Intensity of renal support in critically ill patients with acute kidney injury. N Engl J Med 2008; 359(1):7-20.

Tolwani A. Continuous renal-replacement therapy for acute kidney injury. New Engl J Med 2012;367(26):2505-14.

do Nascimento GV, Gabriel DP, Abrao JM, Balbi AL. When is dialysis indicated in acute kidney injury? Ren Fail 2010;32(3):396-400."

13 Chronic Kidney Disease (CKD)

13.1 Introduction

This chapter will discuss the clinical management of chronic kidney disease (CKD). That will include the following:
- Methods to measure or estimate renal function
- Staging of CKD
- Treatment to slow the progression of kidney dysfunction
- CKD complications and management (specifically, anemia, mineral metabolism, and bone disease, while other issues such as HTN will be discussed elsewhere)
- Cardiovascular disease risk and prevention in CKD patients
- Preparations for renal replacement therapy

13.2 Stages of CKD (according to K/DOQI 2002 clinical practice guidelines)

CKD Stage	Description Findings present for ≥ 3 months	GFR (mL/min/ 1.73 m^2)
Stage 1	Kidney damage with normal or relatively high GFR Kidney damage is defined as pathologic abnormalities or markers of damage, including abnormalities in blood or urine test or imaging studies	≥90
Stage 2	Kidney damage with mild reduction in GFR	60-89
Stage 3	Moderate reduction in GFR	30-59
Stage 4	Severe reduction in GFR. Preparation for renal replacement therapy	15-29
Stage 5	Established kidney failure, that includes end-stage renal disease (defined as a need for renal replacement therapy, ie, dialysis or kidney transplantation)	<15

K/DOQI clinical practice guidelines for chronic kidney disease: evaluation, classification, and stratification. Am J Kidney Dis. Feb 2002;39(2 Suppl 1):S1-266.

13.3 KDIGO Stages of CKD

Although the 2012 KDIGO (Kidney Disease Improving Global Outcomes) guidelines have updated the original 2002 KDOQI (Kidney Disease Outcomes Quality Initiative) guidelines in order to add the recognized risk of albuminuria to eGFR in staging the severity of CKD, many institutions have yet to adopt these added categories. Their rationale has been to maintain the simplicity of the KDOQI stages listed above.

Current Chronic Kidney Disease (CKD) Nomenclature Used by KDIGO

"CKD is defined as abnormalities of kidney structure or function, present for >3 months, with implications for health, and CKD is classified based on cause, GFR category, and albuminuria category" as shown below.

Prognosis of CKD by GFR & Albuminuria Category

Prognosis of CKD by GFR and Albuminuria Catergories: KDIGO 2012			Persistent albuminuria categories Description and range		
			A1	A2	A3
			Normal to mildly increased	Moderately increased	Severely increased
			<30 mg/g <3 mmol	30–300 mg/g 3–30 mmol	>300 mg/g >3 mmol
GFR categories (ml/min.1.73m²) Description and range	G1	Normal or high	≥ 90		
	G2	Mildly decreased	60–89		
	G3a	Mildly to moderately decreased	45–59		
	G3b	Moderately to severely decreased	30–44		
	G4	Severely decreased	15–29		
	G5	Kidney failure	<15		

Green: low risk (if no other markers of kidney disease, no CKD); Yellow: moderately increased risk; Orange: high risk; Red, very high risk.

KDIGO 2012 Clinical Practice Guideline for the Evaluation and Management of Chronic Kidney Disease.

KDIGO "recommends referral to specialist kidney care services for people with CKD" in the following circumstances:

- AKI or abrupt sustained fall in GFR
- GFR <30 ml/min/1.73 m^2 or GFR categories G4-G5
- A consistent finding of significant albuminuria (ACR ≥300 mg/g [≥30 mg/mmol] or AER ≥300 mg/24 hours, approximately equivalent to PCR ≥500 mg/g [≥50 mg/mmol] or PER ≥500 mg/24 hours)
- Progression of CKD - defined based on one of more of the following:
  - Decline in GFR - A certain drop in eGFR is defined as a drop in GFR category (eg, G1 to G2) accompanied by a 25% or greater drop in eGFR from baseline.
  - Rapid progression defined as a sustained decline in eGFR of more than 5 ml/min/1.73 m^2
- Urinary red cell casts, RBC >20/hpf sustained and not readily explained
- CKD and hypertension refractory to treatment with 4 or more antihypertensive agents
- Persistent abnormalities of serum potassium
- Recurrent or extensive nephrolithiasis
- Hereditary kidney disease.

Note: ACR = albumin creatinine ratio; AER = albumin excretion rate; PCR = protein creatinine ratio; PER = protein excretion rate

KDIGO "recommends timely referral for planning renal replacement therapy (RRT) in people with progressive CKD in whom the risk of kidney failure within 1 year is 10–20% or higher, as determined by validated risk prediction tools" as shown below.

Referral to Specialist Services

				Persistent albuminuria categories Description and range		
				A1	A2	A3
				Normal to mildly increased	Moderately increased	Severely increased
				<30 mg/g <3 mg/mmol	30–300 mg/g 3–30 mg/mmol	>300 mg/g >3 mg/mmol
GFR categories (ml/min.1.73m²) Description and range	G1	Normal or high	≥ 90		Monitor	Refer*
	G2	Mildly decreased	60–89		Monitor	Refer*
	G3a	Mildly to moderately decreased	45–59	Monitor	Monitor	Refer*
	G3b	Moderately to severely decreased	30–44	Monitor	Monitor	Refer*
	G4	Severely decreased	15–29	Refer*	Refer*	Refer*
	G5	Kidney failure	<15	Refer*	Refer*	Refer*

Referral decision making by GFR and albuminuria. *Referring clinicians may wish to discuss with their nephrology service depending on local arrangements regarding monitoring or referring.

13.4   Equations – To Calculate GFR Based on Serum Creatinine (S_{Cr})

Cockcroft-Gault equation (to calculate estimated creatinine clearance)

Estimated creatinine clearance (eC_{Cr}):

$$eC_{Cr} \text{ (ml/min)} = \frac{(140 - age)}{S_{Cr} \text{ (mg/dL)}} \times \frac{\text{Body weight (Kg)}}{72} \times (0.85 \text{ if female})$$

where age is expressed in years, SCr in mg/dL, and weight in Kg (original formula used actual weight, now ideal body weight is usually used because of erroneously high results in obese persons). The Cockcroft-Gault equation is still used for some pharmacologic dosing purposes, but has been largely replaced by one of the MDRD eGFR equations or its updated form, the CKD-EPI equation, which is more accurate and doesn't require body weight.

Chronic Kidney Disease Epidemiology Collaboration (CKD-EPI) expression

This expression is considered to be the most accurate estimate of GFR and is advised by the KDIGO guidelines. Since the formulae shown below aren't easy to use in practice, calculators are available on various websites or mobile calculators. The National Kidney Foundation eGFR calculator website is http://www.kidney.org/professionals/kdoqi/gfr.cfm

Race and Sex	Serum Creatinine μmol/L (mg/dL)	Equation
Black		
Female	≤62 (≤0.7)	GFR = 166 × (Scr/0.7)$^{-0.329}$ × (0.993)^{Age}
	>62 (>0.7)	GFR = 166 × (Scr/0.7)$^{-1.209}$ × (0.993)^{Age}
Male	≤80 (≤0.9)	GFR = 163 × (Scr/0.9)$^{-0.411}$ × (0.993)^{Age}
	>80 (>0.9)	GFR = 163 × (Scr/0.9)$^{-1.209}$ × (0.993)^{Age}
White or other		
Female	≤62 (≤0.7)	GFR = 144 × (Scr/0.7)$^{-0.329}$ × (0.993)^{Age}
	>62 (>0.7)	GFR = 144 × (Scr/0.7)$^{-1.209}$ × (0.993)^{Age}
Male	≤80 (≤0.9)	GFR = 141 × (Scr/0.9)$^{-0.411}$ × (0.993)^{Age}
	>80 (>0.9)	GFR = 141 × (Scr/0.9)$^{-1.209}$ × (0.993)^{Age}

13.4.1　Problems with using estimated GFR

- Creatinine, a product of the metabolism of creatine and phosphocreatine in skeletal muscle, is not specific to kidney function. Creatinine will be increased with higher production, as in African-Americans, and decreased in Hispanics and Asians (as compared to Whites). It will be normally higher in younger people with higher muscle mass, higher in males compared to females, and will depend on diet, eg, will be lower in vegetarians.
- In addition to glomerular filtration, creatinine has some renal tubular secretion. Certain medications can decrease tubular secretion that will increase the serum creatinine (eg, trimethoprim, cimetidine), some may increase its measurement (flucytosine, cephalosporins, and perhaps tenofovir), while others may decrease it (eg, methyldopa, ethamsylate)
- Creatinine assay is not consistent between different laboratories and needs to be calibrated
- Poor performance of the equations in some patient populations: Very old and very young, normal and very low renal function, very large and very small individuals, and variable in kidney transplant recipients.

13.4.2　Methods to analyze GFR

	Advantages	Problems/Disadvantages
Creatinine clearance based on 24 hour urine collection	Easy to do, creatinine is an endogenous product	Inaccurate collection by patient, tends to overestimate GFR (because of tubular secretion of creatinine)
Mean of urea and creatinine clearance	Might be more accurate than creatinine clearance, especially in advanced renal insufficiency	Same problem as above
Cystatin C (serum measurement)	A protein from all nucleated cells that undergoes glomerular filtration with reabsorption and catabolism by renal tubular cells.	High variability of serum level between patients. Not very specific (levels are increased) in malignancy, HIV, steroid therapy
Inulin clearance	"Gold standard" (a 5200 dalton polymer of fructose)	Inulin is difficult to measure and a time-consuming, expensive method

cont.	Advantages	Problems/Disadvantages
Radioisotopic methods (eg, 99mTc-labeled diethylene-triaminopentacetic acid (DTPA), 51Cr-EDTA, 125I-iothalamate)	Easy to perform, accurate	Not readily available, require infusion of the radionuclide, radioactive precautions, material is expensive, cannot use it in pregnancy, less accurate in advanced renal failure
Radiocontrast agents (eg, iothalamate, diatrizoate, iohexol)	Accurate and easy to perform	Require infusion of the contrast agent

13.6 Equations – To Calculate GFR Based on Serum Cystatin C or Creatinine & Cystatin

Since studies indicate that serum levels of cystatin C may offer a better estimate of eGFR and of adverse outcomes than creatinine, a CKD-EPI cystatin formula is as follows:

$$eGFR = 133 \times \min(Scys/0.8, 1)^{-0.499} \times \max(Scys/0.8, 1)^{-1.328} \times 0.996^{age} \times [\times 0.932 \text{ if female}]$$

where Scys is serum cystatin C, min indicates the minimum of Scr/κ or 1, and max indicates the maximum of Scys/κ or 1.

The use of combining both serum markers, creatinine and cystatin C, into a single CKD-EPI creatinine-cystatin C equation as shown below appears to offer still better accuracy.

$$eGFR = 135 \times \min(Scr/\kappa, 1)^{\alpha} \times \max(Scr/\kappa, 1)^{-0.601} \times \min(Scys/0.8, 1)^{-0.375} \times \max(Scys/0.8, 1)^{-0.711} \times 0.995^{age} \times [\times 0.969 \text{ if female}] \times [\times 1.08 \text{ if black}]$$

where Scr is serum creatinine, Scys is serum cystatin C, κ is 0.7 for females and 0.9 for males, α is -0.248 for females and -0.207 for males, min indicates the minimum of Scr/κ or 1, and max indicates the maximum of Scr/κ or 1.

From Inker LA, Schmid CH, Tighiouart H, et al. Estimating glomerular filtration rate from serum creatinine and cystatin C. N Engl J Med Jul 5 2012;367(1):20-9.
A website offering a simple calculator for the above equations is available at: http://www.nephromatic.com/egfr.php

13.7 Aging Kidney

Aging Kidney

Physiologic changes with aging

- Enhanced sensitivity to vasoconstrictor stimuli and decreased vasodilatory capacity
- Systemic renin-angiotensin system is suppressed but intrarenal renin-angiotensin system is not
- Prolonged low levels of renin and aldosterone
  → exaggerated renal response to renin-angiotensin system
- Decrease in NO → increased renal vasoconstriction, sodium retention, matrix production and mesangial fibrosis
- Reduced cardiac output, systemic hypertension → ↓ renal perfusion (reduced renal plasma flow ~10% per decade) and ↓ glomerular filtration
- Increases in cellular oxidative stress → endothelial cell dysfunction and changes in vasoactive mediators → increased atherosclerosis, hypertension and glomerulosclerosis
- Cell senescence in the aging kidney

Senile morphological changes

Glomerular
- Glomerulosclerosis
- Mesangial expansion
- Folding & thickening of GBM
- GBM condenses into hyaline material with glomerular tuft collapse

Vascular changes
- Atherosclerosis
- Vascular dysautonomia
- Arteriole subendothelial hyaline & collagen deposits & intimal thickening
- Aglomerular circulation (direct flow betw. afferent & efferent arterioles)

Tubulo-interstitial changes
- Tubular diverticuli
- Tubular atrophy
- Tubular fat degeneration
- Interstitial fibrosis

Reduced renal mass, primarily cortical, with relative sparing of the medulla

Functional changes

- Reduced GFR (from the age of approximately 30 years old, GFR declines at approximately 8 ml/min/1.73 m^2 per decade) accompanied by decreased muscular creatinine production resulting in relatively stable serum Cr
- Medullary hypotonicity → inability to maximally concentrate the urine as well
- Diminished urinary dilution capability
- Diminished plasma renin and aldosterone → reduced sodium reabsorption (increased fractional excretion of Na) and potassium secretion

13.7.1 Differences between a kidney aging normally and a kidney with CKD

Based on reduced estimated GFR below 60 ml/min/1.73 m², many healthy elderly are diagnosed with CKD, but with normal aging:

- Proximal tubular function is preserved
- Serum erythropoietin and hemoglobin levels are normal
- Urea reabsorption is decreased and serum urea level is normal, whereas it is increased in CKD
- Normal levels of calcium, magnesium, phosphate, PTH, and vitamin D
- Normal urinalysis (no hematuria or proteinuria); however, ↓ urinary creatinine excretion in the elderly leads to an elevated urine albumin/creatinine ratio
- Renal reserve (the capacity of the kidney to increase its basal GFR by at least 20% after an adequate stimulus such as a protein load) is preserved in the elderly although the magnitude is decreased

13.8 Management of patient with CKD/ESRD

- Treatment of underlying disease, (eg, control of diabetes, immunosuppression of SLE)
- HTN (targets are not completely clear, but generally <140/90 for uncomplicated HTN, <130/85 for diabetes or renal disease, <125/75 with proteinuria >1 g/day)
- Use of renin-angiotensin inhibition or angiotensin receptor blockers with proteinuria (see 10.7 Hypertension treatment →162)
- Anemia (address need for EPO, iron, and additional work-up)
- Metabolic bone disease (Ca, phosphate, PTH, vitamin D)
- Nutrition (albumin, pre-albumin, vitamins, consider protein restriction of 0.8 mg/kg/d)
- Volume status and sodium restriction or diuretic use
- Acid-base state (eg, bicarbonate supplementation for metabolic acidosis)
- Lipid control for prevention of the increased risk of CV disease
- Adjust medications for decreased GFR (eg, consider stopping metformin) and avoid potential nephrotoxins (NSAIDs)
- Potential for preemptive transplantation (refer when GFR is <20 ml/min)
- Options counseling for renal replacement modality, eg, peritoneal dialysis, incenter hemodialysis, or home hemodialysis
- Creation of vascular access when hemodialysis is elected (establish access when GFR <20 ml/min or Cr >4 mg/dL or dialysis is anticipated in 6 months)
- Dialysis and renal transplant management are discussed in a later chapter.

13.9 Anemia

13.9.1 Workup

Initiate anemia workup
- Hb <11 g/dL or Hct <33% in pre-menopausal females and pre-pubertal patients
- Hb <12 g/dL or Hct <37% in adult males and post-menopausal females

Initial workup of anemia in CKD
- Hb/Hct
- RBC indices, particularly MCV
- Reticulocyte count
- Iron studies
  - Serum iron (reflects iron immediately available for Hb synthesis); measured serum iron = iron bound to transferrin
  - Transferrin = total iron binding capacity or TIBC, either of which can be measured directly or calculated from the other
  - Percent transferrin saturation or TSAT (reflects iron immediately available for Hb synthesis: TSAT <20 % suggests iron deficiency): Calculate TSAT = (Iron/TIBC) x 100%. TSAT indicates how many transferrin binding sites are occupied by iron
  - Serum ferritin (reflects iron stores: normal 40-200 ng/ml, <15 ng/ml makes iron deficiency most likely; a rise to >100 ng/ml is suggestive of a response to iron supplementation)
- Stool for occult blood
- Vitamin B_{12} and folate
- Corrected reticulocytes - what reticulocyte % would be if patient was not anemic: corrected reticulocytes = (Hct/45) x patient's reticulocytes
- Hepcidin, increased in inflammatory states and CKD, interferes with intestinal iron uptake and utilization, but is not yet measured clinically
- If no other cause for anemia is found and serum creatinine is >2 mg/dL, anemia is more likely to be secondary to CKD and relative erythropoietin (EPO) deficiency

13.9.2 Causes of anemia

The following diagram shows potential causes of anemia. It is applicable not only to patients with CKD, but to patients with normal kidney function as well. It is important to remember that CKD patients may have anemia due to factors unrelated to CKD itself, such as blood loss or hemolysis. Although EPO deficiency is a primary cause of anemia in dialysis patients, a lot of other physiologic factors can interfere with erythropoiesis (iron deficiency, inflammation and infection, elevated hepcidin levels, vitamin deficiency, protein malnutrition, hyperparathyroidism, malignancies, and hematologic disorders). .

Causes of Anemia

Initial approach is based on three studies:
Reticulocyte count, MCV, and peripheral smear

Reticulocyte count
- Low if ↓ RBC production (aplastic or hypoplastic anemia)
- High if ↑ RBC production due to ↑ destruction/loss (hemolysis, blood loss)

M C V

Peripheral smear abnormalities
- Spherocytes (AIHA, hereditary spherocytosis)
- Schistocytes indicate microangiopathic hemolysis (TTP/HUS, HELLP, DIC, vasculitis)
- Heart valve hemolysis
- Target cells (alcoholics with liver disease, hemoglobinopathies)
- Teardrops (myelofibrosis)
- Hypersegmented PMNs (B₁₂ deficiency)

Low
- **Iron deficiency:** ↑TIBC/ transferrin, ↓ serum iron, ↓ ferritin, ↓ transferrin saturation (NI or ↓ retics)
- **Chronic disease:** ↓TIBC, ↓ or NI serum iron, ↑ or NI ferritin, ↓ transferrin saturation
- Thalassemi (↑retic count)
- Sideroblastic: Disorders of heme synthesis (NI or ↓ retics)
- Lead poisoning
- Paroxsmal nocturnal hemoglobinuria (↑ retic count)
- **Aluminum excess**

Normal
- **Chronic disease** (chronic inflammation, chronic infection, neoplasms – increased cytokines suppress EPO production and erythropoiesis): ↓ iron, TIBC, NI to ↑ ferritin
- **Renal failure** (↓EPO); anemia of CRF = relative EPO deficiency
- Hypothyroidism
- Aplastic anemia
- Combination of macro- & microcytic causes
- Hemolytic anemia
- **Severe hyperparathyroidism**

High
- Megaloblastic: Hypersegmentation of neutrophils (Impaired DNA synthesis: B₁₂ or folate deficiency, myelodysplastic syndrome, anti-cancer meds)
- Non-megaloblastic (↑ reticulocyte count/ hemolysis/blood loss, **iron excess, EPO treatment**, alcoholism, liver disease, hypothyroidism, smoking, aplastic anemia)

The conditions listed in **bold letters** are causes of anemia more specific to the CKD

13.9.3 Differential diagnosis of causes of anemia

Differential diagnosis of common causes of anemia in CKD: Iron deficiency, erythropoietin deficiency and anemia of chronic disease based on iron studies

	Iron Deficiency	Anemia of CRF	Anemia of Chronic Disease
Iron and TSAT	↓	Nl	↓ or Nl
Total iron binding capacity (TIBC)	↑	Nl	↓ or Nl
Ferritin and bone marrow iron storages	↓	Nl	↑ or Nl
Treatment	Iron supplement (may require IV iron, if oral is unsuccessful)	EPO	Treat the cause, if untreatable, eg, HIV/AIDS - EPO unless its effect to increase cancer growth is a contraindication

TSAT: Transferrin saturation; **TIBC:** Total iron binding capacity; **EPO:** Erythropoietin

13.9.4 Treatment of Anemia of CRF

Iron Therapy

<u>Goal:</u> Maintain TSAT ≥ 20%, ferritin ≥ 100 ng/ml

↓

Monitoring iron (TSAT and ferritin)

- During initiation of EPO Rx and ↑EPO dose check TSAT and ferritin
  - Every 1–2 months when not on IV iron
  - Every 3 months when on IV iron supplementation
- After target Hb is achieved – every 3 months
- In CKD not on EPO with TSAT ≥ 20% and ferritin ≥ 100 ng/ml
  - Every 3–6 months

Oral iron Tx	IV iron therapy	Intramuscular administration

<u>Daily dose:</u>
• At least 200 mg of elemental iron in adults
• 2–3 mg/kg in children
<u>Problems:</u>
• Low intestinal absorption
• Low compliance
  - Inconvenience of dosing
  - Side effects (gastric irritation, constipation)
  - Out-of-pocket expenses
	<u>Administration forms:</u>
	• Iron dextran, iron sucrose, sodium ferric gluconate, ferumoxytol
	<u>Doses:</u>
	• For replacement, doses of 100–125 mg administered at hemodialysis every other day or 300–510 mg every 7–14 days (product dependent) to a total loading dose of 1000 mg elemental iron.
	• For prevention of iron deficiency on hemodialysis, 25–125 mg every week have been used as maintenance therapy, following ferritin levels.
		Iron dextran (rarely used I.M.)
		<u>Problems:</u>
		• Injections are painful and can leave a brownish discoloration
		• Risk of bleeding into the muscle
		• Reports of muscle sarcomas at the site of injection
		• Absorption and bioavailability highly variable

IV Iron Administration & Monitoring of Response

IV iron therapy when TSAT <20% and ferritin <100 ng/ml:

1000 mg of IV iron (see above chart) with repeat if poor response and persistent TSAT < 20% and ferritin <100 ng/ml

Good response when Hb rises to goal and TSAT >20% and ferritin >100 ng/ml:	Hb still low but iron replaced to goal (TSAT >20% and ferritin >100 ng/ml):
For non-HD CKD, follow TSAT & ferritin; maintenance dose iron of 25–125 mg/wk for HD losses of iron in dialysis	Consider ↑EPO dose and another course of 1000 mg IV iron

If Hb remains low, but ↑TSAT or ferritin:
- Reduce iron to lowest dose required to maintain TSAT ≥20% and ferritin ≥100 ng/ml
- If TSAT ≥50% and ferritin ≥800–1200 ng/ml – unlikely to respond to iron – withhold iron, re-measure TSAT and ferritin in 3 months, if ↓ to <50% and <800 ng/ml, resume maintenance IV iron at 1/2–2/3 of initial dose

13.10 EPO Therapy

13.10.1 Indications

- Anemia associated with CKD with no other cause found and when iron deficiency has been corrected with iron Rx
- Also for treatment of anemia in patients treated with zidovudine for HIV infection, scheduled to undergo elective surgery to reduce the need for blood transfusion.

  Patients with cancer on chemotherapy require a risk: benefit assessment in the use of EPO due to finding increased deaths in those with cancer.

13.10.2 Route of EPO administration

- SC - predialysis and PD patients
- IV in HD patients for comfort or SC for better dose response

13.10.3 If switching from IV to SC administration in HD Patients

- If Hb target not yet achieved: SC dose = IV dose
- If at Hb target: SC dose = 2/3 IV dose
- If switching to IV dose = 1.5 SC dose

13.10.4 EPO Dosing

- Epoetin (alfa in the USA) SC in adults 80-120 U/Kg/wk (~6,000U/wk) in 2-3 doses
- Epoetin (alfa in the USA) IV in HD 120-180 U/Kg/wk (~9,000U/wk) in three doses
- If failed to ↑ Hb by 0.5-1.0 g/dL over 2-4 wks - increase EPO dose by 50%
- If Hb ↑ by >1.5 g/dL per month or if Hb exceeds target - reduce weekly dose by 25% (if rapid responder stop and restart 1-2 wks later at 75% of original dose)
- Aim to achieve a target Hb within 2 to 4 month period

13.10.5 EPO controversy

No benefit (CREATE study) and possible cardiovascular harm (CHOIR study) of higher Hb target >12 g/dl (outcome: composite death and cardiovascular events).
No patient event-free survival benefit to having an Hb level of 12.5 g/dl over 10.6 g/dL, but more strokes and more cancer deaths in a subset of patients with previous malignancy, more venous and arterial thromboses (TREAT study).
Risk for mortality is the same from an Hb of 10.0 g/dL up to 12.0 g/dl (DOPPS study).

13.11 Mineral & Bone Disease in CKD

Mineral and bone disease in CKD usually refers to the complex multisystem disorder that involves imbalance of calcium and phosphate, metabolic acidosis, parathyroid dysfunction, vitamin D deficiency, renal osteodystrophy and vascular calcification. We will primarily focus on three aspects that receive most of the attention in clinical practice of nephrology and largely overlap: Controlling hyperphosphatemia, hyperparathyroidism, and renal osteodystrophy.

13.11.1 Cellular components of the bone and their regulation

Osteoblasts
Function
Derived from mesenchymal stem cells, osteoblasts produce collagen and noncollagen proteins on the bone surface to create a structure for mineralization (matrix). Some of the osteoblasts are buried in the matrix and become osteocytes, some become lining cells that line most trabecular bone surfaces and separate the bone from marrow space.
Regulation
Osteoblasts receptors: For PTH, calcitriol (1,25-dihydroxyvitamin D), glucocorticoids, sex hormones, growth hormone (GH) and thyroid hormone, IL-1, TNFa, prostaglandins, insulin-like growth factors (IGFs), transforming growth factor (TGF)-beta, bone morphogenic proteins, fibroblast growth factors, and platelet-derived growth factor.
Factors produced by osteoblasts that probably act locally include prostaglandins, IL-6, IGFs and their binding proteins (IGF-BPs), TGF-beta, bone morphogenic proteins, fibroblast growth factors, platelet-derived growth factor, and vascular-endothelial growth factor.

Osteoclasts
Function
• Related to monocyte/macrophage cells, osteoclasts resorb bone by dissolving mineral and degrading matrix • Excessive osteoclastic resorption occurs in osteoporosis, Paget's disease, hyperparathyroidism and inflammatory bone loss • Inadequate resorption causes osteopetrosis
Regulation
• Many hormones and local factors also can act on osteoblasts to promote or inhibit osteoclastogenesis • Stimulators: Calcitriol, PTH, TNF alpha, prostaglandin E2, IL-1, IL-11, and IL-6 • Inhibitors are IL-4, IL-13 and interferon-gamma (IFNg)

13.11.2 Calcium – phosphate metabolism in CKD

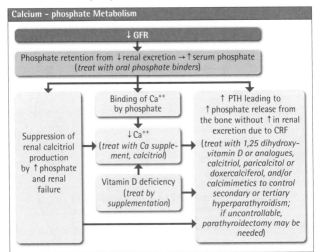

13.11.3 Role of hyperphosphatemia in CKD bone disease, progression and comorbidities

Role of Hyperphosphatemia

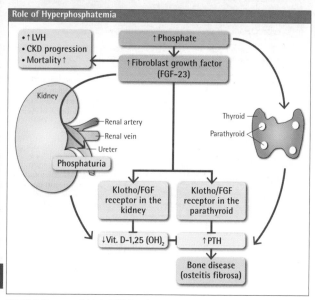

13.11.4 Causes of high PTH level

- Hypocalcemia
- Decreased calcitriol activity
- Decreased sensitivity to Ca by parathyroid calcium-sensing receptor
- Hyperphosphatemia
- Skeletal resistance to the calcemic action of PTH
- Metabolic acidosis
- May develop autonomous tertiary hyperparathyroidism

13.11.5 Forms of hyperparathyroidism

Type of Hyperparathyroidism	Mechanism
Primary: Primary hyperparathyroidism: adenoma (85%), hyperplasia (15%), or carcinoma (<1%) of the parathyroid glands	Primary elevated PTH production
Secondary	Elevated PTH secondary to other factors (low Ca^{++} levels, vitamin D deficiency, renal failure) causing ↑ PTH
Tertiary: Development of autonomous (hypercalcemic) hyperparathyroidism after a period of secondary (normocalcemic or hypocalcemic) hyperparathyroidism with an underlying cause such as malabsorption syndrome or chronic renal failure	After long standing secondary hyperparathyroidism (b/o prolonged over-stimulation of parathyroid gland - may develop adenoma or severe hyperplasia, now with persistent elevated Ca^{++})
Pseudohyperparathyroidism	Elevated PTH with resistance in end-organs causing hypocalcemia

13.11.6 Therapeutic options for secondary hyperparathyroidism

- **Phosphate binders**
  - When GFR is 25% of normal - most patients require limitation of phosphate intake and oral phosphate binders to maintain the serum phosphate below a normal level of 4.5 mg/dl.
  - Calcium salts (risk of hypercalcemia, calciphylaxis, and vascular calcification), eg, calcium carbonate (acetate, carbonate, citrate) (start with 1-2 500-mg pills with each meal, usually require 5-15 g/d) - hypercalcemia (serum Ca >10.2 mg/dl)s is a side effect (correct with lower dialysate Ca to 2.5 mEq/L or less)
  - Calcium-free binders (sevelamer, lanthanum carbonate) reduce phosphate without increasing Ca level, but do not significantly reduce PTH
  - Aluminum containing compounds (cause accumulation of aluminium in brain and bone) - may use for brief courses if Ca x Phos solubility product >65
  - Mg containing antacids - may induce hypermagnesemia and cause diarrhea
- **Vitamin D and vitamin D analogues** (activate vitamin D receptor of parathyroid)
  - Calcitriol, paricalcitol, doxercalciferol, alfacalcidol, 22-oxacalcitriol
  - Risk: Hypercalcemia, hyperphosphatemia, excessive suppression of PTH
  - Should not be used in hypercalcemia or hyperphosphatemia (when Ca x Phos solubility product >70) - will increase intestinal absorption of Ca and Phos, exacerbating Ca x Phos solubility product

Therapeutic options for secondary hyperparathyroidism
Vitamin D and vitamin D analogues (cont.)
- For PTH suppression - goal: Decrease PTH to 2-3 times normal (to about 150-300 pg/ml in stage 5 CKD to decrease risk of osteitis fibrosa, yet not induce adynamic bone osteodystrophy).
- Vitamin D analogues (eg, paricalcitol), selective for PTH receptors, might affect intestinal receptors and Ca/phos absorption to a lesser extent than calcitriol lessening rise of serum Ca and phos

- **Calcimimetics**
  - Activate/upregulate Ca-sensing receptor of parathyroid (eg, cinacalcet)
  - May inhibit parathyroid hyperplasia
  - Side effect: hypocalcemia (managed with dose adjustment or vitamin D administration)

- **Bisphosphonates** (limiting the high rate of bone resorption) as a bridge to more definitive treatment of secondary hyperparathyroidism or as a treatment for osteoporosis, should be used selectively and with caution when eGFR <30 ml/min

- **Parathyroidectomy** in severe hyperparathyroidism, when medical treatment has failed

- **Other methods**
  - Percutaneous parathyroid injection of ethanol or vitamin D compounds
  - Correct acidosis
  - Estrogen supplements for osteoporosis (has risk of increased thrombosis)

13.11.7 Indications for Parathyroidectomy
Uncontrolled levels of PTH + hypercalcemia + complications:

- Osteitis fibrosa
- Extraskeletal calcification
- Calciphylaxis
- Persistent serum Ca >11.5 mg/dl
- Persistent uncontrollable hyperphosphatemia
- Skeletal pain or fractures
- Intractable pruritus

Effect of parathyroidectomy

- Improved PTH
- Improved Ca
- Improved anemia
- Improved BP control
- May improve intractable pruritus

13.11.8 Renal osteodystrophy

High Turnover Bone Disease (↑ PTH)	Low Turnover Bone Disease (↓ PTH)
Osteitis fibrosa (↑ osteoclast number, size, and activity, ↑ bone resorption, marrow fibrosis, ↑ osteoblastic activity), deposition of collagen is less ordered, ↑ rate of bone formation, and ↑ unmineralized bone matrix (osteoid)	• **Osteomalacia:** Reductions in bone turnover, the number of bone-forming and bone-resorbing cells, and an increase in the osteoid formation and volume of unmineralized bone (the rate of mineralization is slower than collagen synthesis). **Causes :** Vitamin D deficiency, aluminum intoxication, long standing metabolic acidosis • **Adynamic/aplastic bone lesions:** Reduced bone turnover, no increase in osteoid formation (↓ mineralization, but normal amount of osteoid). **Causes:** Aluminum deposition (in a minority of cases), oversuppression of PTH, calcitriol may directly suppress osteoblastic activity, use of oral Ca carbonate.

13.11.9 Osteoporosis management in CKD

Diagnosis
Bone loss in osteoporosis compared with age-matched group (Z-score) and young group (T-score): • 0 - 1 standard deviations about the mean - normal • 1 - 2.5 standard deviations below - osteopenia • >2.5 standard deviations below - osteoporosis

Treatment
Treatment nonspecific for CKD
• Estrogen replacement • Calcitonin • Bisphosphonate (alendronate) use selectively and with caution in patients with CKD
Treatment specific for CKD
• Treat hyperparathyroidism and hyperphosphatemia • Correct metabolic acidosis

13.12 Uremic Coagulopathy

As part of the uremic complications of severe renal failure, patients may develop bleeding. The coagulopathy is associated with diminished platelet adhesion and aggregation which may be manifested by a prolonged bleeding time. Multiple mechanisms related to circulating uremic toxins, anemia, vascular and platelet metabolic abnormalities of arachidonic acid metabolism, and defects in Factor VIII complex and von Willebrand factor activity may play a role in the diminished platelet, fibrinogen and vascular endothelial binding. Since dialysis only slowly reverses these defects, treatment with DDAVP or cryoprecipitate which elevate Factor VIII and von Willebrand factor is the mainstay of treatment when bleeding in uremic patients is active or anticipated.

13.12.1 Treatment of Uremic Coagulopathy

Treatment	Peak Action	Duration
DDAVP, 0.3 µg/Kg IV in 50 ml over 15 min (or SC)	1 hour	4–8 hours
Cryoprecipitate, 7–10 units IV	2–4 hours	12–24 hours
Conjugated estrogens, 0.6 mg/Kg IV or orally daily for 5 days	1–5 days	Up to 14 days
Dialysis	Days	Indefinite
EPO (+ iron prn) to Hct >30% (may have a beneficial effect)	Days	Indefinite

13.13 Nutrition & Role of Low Protein Diet

The role of protein restriction in progression of CKD remains controversial and evidence for use of protein restriction is inconclusive. However, if there is no safety concern regarding potential malnutrition, this maneuver can be implemented, often improving early uremic symptoms such as anorexia. While urea itself is not a toxic compound, other byproducts of protein metabolism might lead to CKD progression, eg, asymmetric dimethylarginine (ADMA).

13.13.1 Nutritional needs

	Sufficient Protein Intake	Calorie Intake
Pre-ESRD patients	0.6-0.8 g/Kg/day (increase to compensate for urinary protein losses)	35 kcal/kg/day
Adult HD patient	1.2 g/Kg/day	35 kcal/kg/day
Adult PD patient	1.3 g/Kg/day (needed for peritoneal protein loss)	35 kcal/kg/day

As CKD progresses, restriction of sodium (<1.5-2 g/day), potassium (<2 g/day), and phosphate (<800 g/day) is usually desirable to prevent edema/ volume overload, hyperkalemia, and hyperphosphatemia, respectively.

13.13.2 Bicarbonate supplementation

Correcting metabolic acidosis to serum HCO_3 >23 mEq/L with oral sodium bicarbonate 0.5-1.0 mEq/Kg/day (usually 2.6-5.2 g/day) or sodium citrate, 1 mEq/ml (30-60 ml/day but citrate may enhance GI absorption of aluminum making it less desirable in severe CKD) helps to avoid bone disease, muscle wasting, anorexia, and may slow progression of CKD.

References and Suggested Reading

CKD evaluation, staging and management

KDIGO 2012 Clinical Practice Guideline for the Evaluation and Management of Chronic Kidney Disease. Kidney Int Suppl Jan 2013; 3(1):1-150.

K/DOQI clinical practice guidelines for chronic kidney disease: evaluation, classification, and stratification. Am J Kidney Dis Feb 2002;39(2 Suppl 1):S1-266.

Fink HA, Ishani A, Taylor BC, et al. Screening for, monitoring, and treatment of chronic kidney disease stages 1to 3: A systematic review for the U.S. Preventive Services Task Force and for the American College of Physicians clinical practice guideline. Ann Intern Med Apr 17 2012;156(8):570-581.

Ruggenenti P, Cravedi P, Remuzzi G. Mechanisms and treatment of CKD. J Am Soc Nephrol Dec 2012; 23(12):1917-1928.

KDIGO clinical practice guideline for the management of blood pressure in chronic kidney disease. Kidney Int Suppl Dec 2012; 2(5): 337-414.

Levey AS. Assessing the effectiveness of therapy to prevent the progression of renal disease. Am J Kidney Di. Jul 1993;22(1):207-214.

Botev R, Mallie JP, Wetzels JF, Couchoud C, Schuck O. The clinician and the estimation of glomerular filtration rate by creatinine-based formulas: current limitations and quo vadis. Clin J Am Soc Nephrol Apr 2011;6(4):937-950.

Traynor J, Mactier R, Geddes CC, Fox JG. How to measure renal function in clinical practice. BMJ Oct 7 2006;333(7571):733-737.

Cockcroft DW, Gault MH. Prediction of creatinine clearance from serum creatinine. Nephron 1976;16(1):31-41.

Levey AS, Bosch JP, Lewis JB, Greene T, Rogers N, Roth D. A more accurate method to estimate glomerular filtration rate from serum creatinine: a new prediction equation. Modification of Diet in Renal Disease Study Group. Ann Intern Med Mar 16 1999;130(6):461-470.

Levey AS, Coresh J, Greene T, et al. Expressing the Modification of Diet in Renal Disease Study equation for estimating glomerular filtration rate with standardized serum creatinine values. Clin Chem Apr 2007;53(4):766-772.

Levey AS, Stevens LA, Schmid CH, et al. A new equation to estimate glomerular filtration rate. Ann Intern Med May 5 2009;150(9):604-612.

Levey AS, Stevens LA. Estimating GFR using the CKD Epidemiology Collaboration (CKD-EPI) creatinine equation: more accurate GFR estimates, lower CKD prevalence estimates, and better risk predictions. Am J Kidney Dis. Apr 2010;55(4):622-627.

Coresh J, Astor BC, McQuillan G, et al. Calibration and random variation of the serum creatinine assay as critical elements of using equations to estimate glomerular filtration rate. Am J Kidney Dis. May 2002;39(5):920-929.

Poggio ED, Wang X, Greene T, Van Lente F, Hall PM. Performance of the modification of diet in renal disease and Cockcroft-Gault equations in the estimation of GFR in health and in chronic kidney disease. J Am Soc Nephrol Feb 2005;16(2):459-466.

Matsushita K, Mahmoodi BK, Woodward M, et al. Comparison of risk prediction using the CKD-EPI equation and the MDRD study equation for estimated glomerular filtration rate. JAMA May 9 2012; 307(18):1941-51.

Inker LA, Schmid CH, Tighiouart H, et al. Estimating glomerular filtration rate from serum creatinine and cystatin C. N Engl J Med Jul 5 2012;367(1):20-9.

Perrone RD, Steinman TI, Beck GJ, et al. Utility of radioisotopic filtration markers in chronic renal insufficiency: simultaneous comparison of 125I-iothalamate, 169Yb-DTPA, 99mTc-DTPA, and inulin. The Modification of Diet in Renal Disease Study. Am J Kidney Dis Sep 1990;16(3):224-235.

References and Suggested Reading (cont.)

Kielstein JT, Fliser D, Veldink H. Asymmetric dimethylarginine and symmetric dimethylarginine: axis of evil or useful alliance? Semin Dial Jul-Aug 2009;22(4):346-350.

Herzog CA, Asinger RW, Berger AK et al. Cardiovascular disease in chronic kidney disease. A clinical update from Kidney Disease: Improving Global Outcomes (KDIGO). Kidney Int 2011; 80: 572-586.

Hering D, Mahfoud F, Walton AS, et al. Renal denervation in moderate to severe CKD. J Am Soc Nephrol 2012; 23:1250-1257.

Fouque D, Laville M. Low protein diets for chronic kidney disease in non-diabetic adults. Cochrane Database Syst Rev 2009: CD001892.

National Kidney Foundation. KDOQI clinical practice guideline for diabetes and chronic kidney disease: 2012 Update. Am J Kidney Dis 2012; 60: 850-886.

deBrito-Ashurst I, Varagunam M, Raftery MJ, Yaqoob MM. Bicarbonate supplementation slows progression of CKD and improves nutritional status. J Am Soc Nephrol (2009 Sep) 20(9):2075-84

The aging kidney

Weinstein JR, Anderson S. The aging kidney: physiological changes. Adv Chronic Kidney Dis 2010; 17: 302-307.

Musso CG, Oreopoulos DG, Aging and physiological changes of the kidneys including changes in glomerular filtration rate, Nephron Physiol 2011; 119 (Suppl 1):1-5.

Yang H, Fogo AB, Cell senescence in the aging kidney, J Am Soc Nephrol 2010; 21:1436-9.

Anemia

KDIGO Anemia Work Group. KDIGO clinical practice guideline for anemia in chronic kidney disease. Kidney Int Suppl 2012; 2: 279-335.

Volkova N, Arab L. Evidence-based systematic literature review of hemoglobin/hematocrit and all-cause mortality in dialysis patients. Am J Kidney Dis Jan 2006;47(1):24-36.

IV. NKF-K/DOQI Clinical Practice Guidelines for Anemia of Chronic Kidney Disease: update 2000. Am J Kidney Dis Jan 2001;37(1 Suppl 1):S182-238.

Port FK, Pisoni RL, Bommer J, et al. Improving outcomes for dialysis patients in the international Dialysis Outcomes and Practice Patterns Study. Clin J Am Soc Nephrol Mar 2006;1(2):246-255.

Macdougall IC. Strategies for iron supplementation: oral versus intravenous. Kidney Int Suppl. Mar 1999;69:S61-66.

Goldsmith D. 2009: a requiem for rHuEPOs--but should we nail down the coffin in 2010? Clin J Am Soc Nephrol May 2010;5(5):929-935.

Drueke TB, Locatelli F, Clyne N, et al. Normalization of hemoglobin level in patients with chronic kidney disease and anemia. N Engl J Med Nov 16 2006;355(20):2071-2084.

Singh AK, Szczech L, Tang KL, et al. Correction of anemia with epoetin alfa in chronic kidney disease. N Engl J Med Nov 16 2006;355(20):2085-2098.

Pfeffer MA, Burdmann EA, Chen CY, et al. A trial of darbepoetin alfa in type 2 diabetes and chronic kidney disease. N Engl J Med Nov 19 2009;361(21):2019-2032.

Goldsmith D, Covic A. Time to Reconsider Evidence for Anaemia Treatment (TREAT) = Essential Safety Arguments (ESA). Nephrol Dial Transplant Jun 2010;25(6):1734-1737.

References and Suggested Reading (cont.)

Mineral, bone and phosphate

KDIGO CKD-MBD Work Group. KDIGO clinical practice guideline for the diagnosis, evaluation, revention, and treatment of Chronic Kidney Disease-Mineral and Bone Disorder (CKD-MBD). Kidney Int Suppl 2009; 76(Suppl 113):S1–130.

Palmer SC, Hayen A, Macaskill P et al. Serum levels of phosphorus, parathyroid hormone, and calcium and risks of death and cardiovascular disease in individuals with chronic kidney disease: a systematic review and meta-analysis. JAMA 2011; 305: 1119–1127.

Eriksen EF. Cellular mechanisms of bone remodeling. Rev Endocr Metab Disord Dec 2010;11(4):219–227.

Cunningham J, Locatelli F, Rodriguez M. Secondary hyperparathyroidism: pathogenesis, disease progression, and therapeutic options. Clin J Am Soc Nephrol Apr 2011;6(4):913–921.

Toussaint ND, Elder GJ, Kerr PG. Bisphosphonates in chronic kidney disease; balancing potential benefits and adverse effects on bone and soft tissue. Clin J Am Soc Nephrol Jan 2009;4(1):221–233.

Kuro OM. Phosphate and Klotho. Kidney Int Suppl Apr 2011(121):S20–23.

Juppner H. Phosphate and FGF-23. Kidney Int Suppl Apr 2011(121):S24–27.

Uremic coagulopathy

Hedges SJ, Dehoney SB, Hooper JS, et al. Evidence-based treatment recommendations for uremic bleeding. Nat Clin Pract Nephrol 2007; 3(3):138-53.

Molino D, De Lucia D, Gaspare De Santo N. Coagulation disorders in uremia. Semin Nephrol Jan 2006; 26(1):46-51.

Jubelirer SJ. Hemostatic abnormalities in renal disease. Am J Kidney Dis May 1985; 5(5):219-25.

14 Dialysis

14.1 Dialysis Initiation

14.1.1 Indications

Indications for initiating dialysis in acute or chronic renal failure are similar — to alleviate symptoms or signs of uremia, abnormalities of electrolyte or acid-base balance, or uncontrolled hypervolemia. Dialysis may be started in severe acute renal failure when no quick recovery is expected to avoid "impending uremia".

14.1.2 Appropriateness of dialysis initiation

• The appropriateness of starting dialysis in a particular patient should be based upon two considerations:
  - Expected patient survival with or without dialysis and
  - Quality of life.
• Elderly patients (>80 years old) with significant co-morbidities might need to be informed that hemodialysis may extend life only 2 – 3 months more than conservative medical management without improving quality of life, although that should be decided individually on a case-by-case basis.

14.1.3 Timing of dialysis initiation

Until recently, there was uncertainty about the timing of dialysis initiation (early vs. late start) in advancing CKD. The definition of early and late was based on the degree of renal dysfunction, measured by creatinine clearance or creatinine-based estimated GFR. But studies have found that there is no benefit to early initiation of dialysis and in fact there is a suggested benefit of a late start based on symptoms or signs of uremia. In acute renal failure there is a suggestion that early initiation of dialysis might be beneficial to patient mortality.

14.2 Indications for Renal Replacement Therapy

Acute Kidney Injury
• Symptoms or signs of the uremic syndrome (pericarditis, seizures, encephalopathy, coagulopathy)
• Refractory hypervolemia, pulmonary edema
• Hyperkalemia
• Acidosis
• Rapidly rising BUN and creatinine with persistent oliguria
• Some poisonings, eg, methanol, ethylene glycol

Chronic Kidney Disease (ESRD)

Absolute

- Uncontrollable hyperkalemia (K^+>6.5 meq/l)
- CHF, fluid overload, and pulmonary edema unresponsive to diuretics
- Uremic symptoms (pericarditis, seizures, progressive neuropathy, encephalopathy, nausea, vomiting, weight loss)
- Significant bleeding with uremic coagulopathy

Relative

- Low GFR 10 ml/min, or <15 ml/min in diabetic, creatinine ≥10 mg/dl. However, estimated GFR should have minor role in determining the time of dialysis initiation
- Intractable HTN with diuretic unresponsiveness in severe CKD

Relative contraindications

- Severe irreversible dementia
- Short estimated survival
- Severe or debilitating co-morbid diseases compromising patient's quality of life

14.3 Dialyzers

Hemodialysis membranes are manufactured with cellulose, modified cellulose, or synthetic polymers. Dialyzer clearance is determined by the surface area (A) and mass transfer coefficient, which is a function of the membrane itself (Ko).

Types of Dialyzers/membranes

- Low flux membranes (standard dialyzers with small pores)
- High efficiency dialyzers (dialyzers with large surface area A)
- High flux dialyzers (increased pore size and increased hydraulic permeability Ko for greater dialysis of "middle" molecules and greater ultrafiltration)
- Protein-leaking membranes (for plasmapheresis to remove large molecules such as immunoglobulins at the price of leaking out albumin)

14.4 Biocompatibility of Dialysis Membrane Interaction with Blood

Alternative Complement Pathway Activation – Generation of C5a

- Mast cell activation with release of histamine and leukotriene – can cause bronchoconstriction and vasodilatation
- Neutrophil activation with degranulation and release of adhesion receptors – can cause endothelial damage, release of β_2-microglobulin
- Monocyte activation, release of IL-1 and TNF-α – can cause hypotension and fever

Factor XII Activation

| Coagulation | Activation of kallikrein |

14.5   Vascular Access for Hemodialysis

There are three main types of vascular access for hemodialysis:
- Arterio-venous fistula (AVF)
- Arterio-venous graft (AVG) and
- Central venous catheter (tunneled or not)

Hemodialysis access should be able to provide a blood flow of at least 300 ml/min.

14.5.1   Types of dialysis access

Arterio–venous fistula

AVF is the preferable dialysis access as it is associated with the best clinical outcomes. It has lower rates of infection, better long-term survival of the patient and of the access itself. However, it requires sufficient vasculature to create an adequate AVF that will mature and be useable to obtain satisfactory blood flow rates. It takes at least 2-3 weeks for an AVF to mature before being used, and more commonly, longer with many fistulae never maturing adequately.

Arterio–venous grafts

AVG is useful in patients where an AVF is not feasible due to poor veins. It provides good blood flow, and because it is internalized, is less prone to infections than a central venous catheter. AVG is considered to be inferior to AVF in terms of patient survival (except in elderly patients with comorbidities). AVG does not require much time to mature and can often be used immediately or within days of placement.

Central venous catheter

CVC is considered to be the last choice for chronic dialysis access, to be used only after AVF and AVG options are not feasible, if there is no time for AVF/AVG maturation, for patients likely to recover from AKI, for patients scheduled for renal transplantation but needing short-term dialysis, or if patient survival is likely to be short. Catheters are associated with poor patient survival, are often complicated by infection, generally have lower blood flow rates, and are more prone to clotting than AVF/AVG. The benefit of a central venous catheter is that it can be used immediately after placement.

14.5.2 Dialysis access monitoring

- Physical exam of pulse and bruit of AVF/AVG
- Venous pressure measurements at dialysis (at blood flow rate (Qb) 200 ml/min, VP should be <130 mm Hg with 15 g needle, <150 mm Hg with 16 g needle)
- Recirculation study when blood flow or dialysis adequacy is poor or every 3 – 6 months
- Blood flow measurements of AVF/AVG followed monthly (though this hasn't been proven effective)

14.5.3 Acute dialysis access

- Double-lumen non-cuffed dialysis catheters (semi-rigid at room temperature to facilitate insertion but soften at body temperature, proximal and distal lumens should be separated by at least 2 cm, max blood flow usually 350-400 ml/min, may be placed in femoral, internal jugular, or less desirably, subclavian veins, (due to high incidence of central vein stenoses) also available with a third lumen for blood sampling or infusions)
- Silastic, cuffed, tunneled dialysis catheters (either double lumen or two single lumen twin catheters usually placed in an internal jugular vein)
- Quinton-Scribner shunts (of historical interest only as these external arteriovenous shunts are not used anymore)

14.5.4 Dialysis catheters

"Ideal" dialysis catheter

- Easy to insert and remove
- Inexpensive
- Low infection rate
- Does not clot or develop fibrin sheath
- Does not cause stenosis of central veins
- Delivers high flow (>400 ml/min) reliably
- Durable material to avoid kinking or leaks
- Comfortable and acceptable to the patient

Duration of catheter use

- Temporary (not tunneled) femoral catheters, inserted with sterile technique and meticulously cleaned daily in bedbound patients, can usually be left in place safely for 3-7 days, occasionally longer, but are not suitable for ambulatory patients
- Subclavian and internal jugular temporary catheters (not tunneled) may be left in place for 2 - 4 weeks.
- Silastic/silicone cuffed catheters (tunneled) are suitable for long-term use

Complications

Dialysis Catheter Complications

Insertion related (ultrasound assistance might help to avoid)

- Pneumothorax
- Hemothorax
- Puncture of a major artery or vein by needle
- Perforation of vein or cardiac chamber by guidewire or catheter
- Pericardial tamponade
- Brachial plexus injury
- Arrhythmia: Transient atrial or ventricular (with insertion of guidewire)
- Air embolism

Later complications

- Infection (see more detailed discussion below)
- Clotting of catheter or formation of a fibrin sheath. Minimize by instillation of heparin, sodium citrate, or tissue plasminogen activator (tPA) following hemodialysis, unproven role of systemic warfarin or low molecular weight heparin, treatment: tPA - 2 mg of tPA (alteplase) into each port will re-establish effective blood flow in 87.5% cases; catheter stripping to remove clot and fibrin sheaths that adhere to the catheter; or exchanging the catheter over a guidewire may be needed
- Central vein thrombosis or stricture (30% - 40% in subclavian, 2% - 10% internal jugular), which may cause loss of use for AVF in ipsilateral arm. DOQI recommends avoidance of subclavian vein unless no other options exist or if the ipsilateral extremity can no longer be used for permanent dialysis access (AVF or AVG) should venous occlusion occur
- IVC thrombosis with lumbar catheter (rarely used unless no other access)
- Arteriovenous fistula formation as rare complication

Infection prophylaxis

- Using tunneled, rather than nontunneled dialysis catheters
- Strict aseptic technique
- The prophylactic use of antibiotics at the time of catheter placement - no effect
- Filling the lumen with antibiotic-anticoagulant after dialysis ("antibiotic lock")
- Treatment of catheter surfaces with minocycline, use of antibiotic-impregnated or silver sulfadiazine-coated catheters (substantial reduction in infection rates)
- Silver-impregnated collagen cuff
- Triple antibiotic ointment or mupirocin ointment to exit site with each dressing change

Treatment

Treatment of Central Venous Catheter-related Infections

Temporary catheter

- Remove catheter
- Antibiotics for 2 weeks

Permanent (tunneled) catheter

1) Exit site infection (catheter removal if Pseudomonas, otherwise antibiotic treatment [ABx] for 1 – 2 wks). Remove catheter if infection persists or systemic signs of sepsis develop

2) Tunnel infection: Catheter removal, surgical drainage, if necessary, ABx for 2 wks

3) Suppurative phlebitis: Remove catheter, Abx for 4 – 6 wks and anticoagulation (old) or thrombolytics (new) or surgical vein excision may be used

4) Bacteremia:
- Gram positive – treat with ABx for 4 weeks (vancomycin for methicillin-resistant organisms): While the catheter remains in place – only 32% of the catheters were successfully salvaged
- Exchange of the catheter over a wire, if no tunnel infection and non-severe symptoms, during a 3 – 4 week course of antibiotics – good initial results, 88% success rate at 45 days
- Bacteremia + exit site or tunnel involvement: Catheter exchange after 24 – 48 h of ABx with creation of new exit site and tunnel with ABx for 4 wks: 75% success rate
- Severe clinical symptoms: Catheter removed, ABx for 4 wks with new catheter placed when bacteremia has cleared: 87% success rate at 45 days
- Immediate catheter removal if bacteremia is caused by:
  - Pseudomonas aeruginosa
  - Vancomycin-resistant enterococcus or staphylococcus
  - Corynebacterium sps
  - Bacillus sps
  - Lactobacillus sps
  - Fungemia
  - Gram positive with bacteremia after 48h of ABx Rx

5) Fever with no identifiable cause (leave catheter in place if there is another source of infection present)

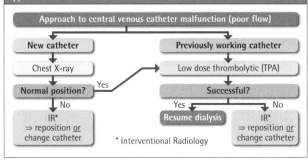

Anticoagulation in hemodialysis

Anticoagulation is an important part of dialysis procedure. Most common options for anticoagulation are unfractionated heparin (United States) and low molecular weight heparin (Western Europe). Other agents are available when heparin is not an option (eg, in heparin-induced thrombocytopenia).

Anticoagulants	Chemical Composition	Mechanism	Follow-up Indicator	Heparin-induced Thrombo-cytopenia
Unfractio-nated heparin	Mixture of glycosaminogly-cane chains 5,000 – 30,000 Da	Binds to anti-thrombin III $\Rightarrow$ inhibits clotting factors IIa and Xa	PTT	1% – 5% incidence
Low molecular weight heparin	Depolymer-ized fragments of larger hep-arins 4,000-6,500 Da	Binds to anti-thrombin III $\Rightarrow$ inhibits clotting factor Xa ($\downarrow$ incidence of bleeding)	Anti-Xa (therapeutic range 0.2 – 0.4 U/ml)	0% – 3% incidence (90% cross reactivity with HIT-IgG)

Anticoagulants (cont.)	Chemical Composition	Mechanism	Follow-up Indicator	Heparin-induced Thrombo-cytopenia
Citrate	Trisodium citrate solution, 3% (ACD-A sol'n) or citrate dialysate	Citrate binds to calcium and disrupts the coagulation cascade	Ionized calcium (therapeutic < 0.4 mM/L in dialyzer) or an activated clotting time of 1.5 - 2.0 times baseline (180 - 250 sec)	None

Other anticoagulants indicated below are usually not used for hemodialysis

Anticoagulants (cont.)	Chemical Composition	Mechanism	Follow-up Indicator	Heparin-induced Thrombo-cytopenia
Heparinoids (danaparoid)	Sulfated glycosaminoglycanes 4,000 - 8,000 Da	Binds to anti-thrombin III ⇒ inhibits clotting factor Xa (incidence of bleeding)	Anti-Xa (therapeutic range 0.2 - 04 U/ml)	0% - 3% incidence (<10% cross reactivity with HIT-IgG)
Hirudin, Lepirudin	Peptide of 65 amino acids	Binds to thrombin	PTT	None
Iloprost	Analogue of prostacyclin	Inhibits platelets aggregation	-	None
Ancrod	Extract from pit viper venom	Cleaves fibrinogen, prevents conversion into the fibrin	-	None

14.6   Hemodialysis adequacy

Determining the adequate dose of dialysis for an individual patient remains uncertain. It is known that adding more dialysis clearance above a certain amount does not continue to provide additional survival benefit. While goals for adequate dialysis dose might change as we learn more, it is important to know the tools to measure dialysis dose. Different approaches to measuring dialysis dose have one common component - the measurement is based on clearance of a particular chemical compound from the blood. Most often urea or creatinine are used as such compounds. Dialysis dose therefore may be expressed as percent reduction in plasma urea concentration (urea reduction ratio or URR). An alternate would be clearance of urea or creatinine in a given time period (Kt = clearance x time) and usually to individualize this indicator to patient size with this calculation based on the patient's total body water volume (V) and expressed as Kt/V. Urea Kt/V and URR are used most often as indicators of hemodialysis dose, while urea Kt/V and creatinine clearance are used as indicators of peritoneal dialysis dose.

Hemodialysis Adequacy	
Urea Reduction Ratio (URR)	**Kt/V (urea)**
$$URR = \frac{(BUN\ predialysis - BUN\ post\ dialysis)}{(BUN\ predialysis)} \times 100\%$$ Minimally adequate URR ≥ 65% for each treatment with three times per week dialysis, though target dose ≥ 70 % is common in patients with little or no residual kidney function	K - clearance of the dialyzer in ml/min, may be calculated from the URR or provided by the manufacturer (eg, at QB = 400 ml/min QD = 800 ml/min, and UF = 15 ml/min urea clearance of the following 3 Fresenius dialyzers, the Optiflux 160NR, Optiflux 200NR, and Gambro Polyflux 210H are approx. 0.28, 0.29, and 0.31 l/min) t - time of dialysis (min) V - volume of distribution of urea based on total body water (ml) Kt - total volume of fluid cleared of urea (ml) Kt/V - how many total body water volumes of distribution of urea are cleared with each dialysis treatment. It can be calculated from URR using empiric formulae or websites such as http://www.kt-v.net/. Minimally adequate Kt/V ≥ 1.2 with three times per week dialysis, though target dose Kt/V ≥1.4 is common, particularly in patients with little or no residual kidney function

14.7 Dialysis drug clearance

Clearance of drugs and pharmacokinetics during hemodialysis is complex. It is important to estimate dialysis clearance of medications to adequately adjust the dose That is especially true in drugs with relatively narrow therapeutic windows (e.g., chemotherapy, antibiotics). The complexity of the process has to do with multiple factors affecting drug clearance in dialysis, specifically, the characteristics of the dialyzer, dialysis procedure, dialysate, and properties of the drug itself. Using these considerations only very crude approximations of the clearance are possible in the absence of experimental data. Such experimental data are obtained for some but not all drugs (eg, vancomycin).

Drug properties that affect dialytic clearance
• Molecular size
- <1000 Da — small molecules — diffusion-dependent transport
- 1000 – 2000 Da — only convective transport
- >2000 Da partially reflected by membrane even during UF
• Protein binding reduces clearance (heparin increases free fraction of many drugs)
• Volume of distribution (the greater the volume of distribution the less the dialyzability)
- 1 L/Kg B.W. distribution volume - likely removed by dialysis
- 1-2 L/Kg B.W distribution volume - marginal clearance by dialysis
- > 2 L/Kg B.W. - unlikely to be effectively removed by dialysis
- Multicompartmental distribution leads to dramatic rebound after dialysis
• Charge of drug molecule
• Water or lipid solubility: Poor dialyzability of lipid-soluble compounds
• Dialyzer membrane binding increases clearance of the compound

Dialysis properties that affect drug clearance
• Dialyzer properties (pore size, surface area, type of membrane might affect binding)
• Dialysis procedure properties (blood flow rate, dialysate flow rate, ultrafiltration rate)
• Dialysate properties (solute concentration, pH, temperature)
• Time of dialysis treatment

14.8 Continuous Renal Replacement Therapy

Indications for the continuous renal replacement therapy (CRRT): need for renal replacement therapy (fluid overload, uremia, uncorrectable acidosis, hyperkalemia, some intoxications) in an hemodynamically unstable patient. CRRT clearance is based on diffusion (dialysis), convection (ultrafiltration), and adsorption by the membrane, similar to clearance by intermittent dialysis though usually less efficient. Most CRRT is done by continuous veno-venous hemofiltration (CVVH), rather than continuous arterio-venous hemofiltration (CAVH), without or with concomitant dialysis, called continuous veno-venous hemodiafiltration (CVVHD).

What do you need to know to write CRRT orders?

Pumps

- Blood flow rate 120–250 (average 180) ml/min
- UF rate 1–2 L/hr total but net UF depends on patient volume status and overall goals of treatment

Replacement fluids

- If standard commercial replacement fluid is not available, normal saline and sodium bicarbonate, peritoneal dialysis fluid, Ringer's lactate, or pharmacy made solutions can be used

Dialysis fluid

- The composition of dialysis fluid is selected based on the same principles as for intermittent hemodialysis; peritoneal dialysate solutions are often used, though calcium-free dialysate may be preferable for citrate anticoagulation.

Anticoagulation

- Systemic heparin or regional citrate anticoagulation
- Citrate anticoagulation
  - ACD-A solution of 3% trisodium citrate infused at a rate of 150% in ml/hr of the blood flow rate (QB) in ml/min, eg, 225 ml/hr for a QB of 150 ml/min
  - Ca^{++} infusion rate is calculated based on the principle of giving about 1 mmol of Ca^{++} for each mmole of citrate, then adjust infusion rate based on ionized calcium (iCa^{++}) level (eg, calcium gluconate 20 g in 500 mL D5W at 30 ml/h with an increase for iCa^{++} <1.0 mmol/L or a decrease for iCa^{++} >1.2 mmol/L)

Parameters to monitor

- Serum electrolytes, iCa^{++}, Mg^{++} Q 4–6 hours
- For citrate anticoagulation, iCa^{++} Q4h initially until stable, then Q6h and total calcium Q12h to assess for citrate toxicity (by an increasing gap between total and ionized calcium levels
- Activated clotting time measured at the post-filter maintained between 180 and 200 seconds with either heparin or citrate is usually adequate

14.9 Peritoneal Dialysis

14.9.1 Techniques

Peritoneal Dialysis Techniques
Manual technique
• CAPD - continuous ambulatory PD (Continuous technique with about four 2–3 liter exchanges per day, 4–6 hours dwell cycles)
Techniques requiring a cycler machine or automated PD (APD)
• CCPD - Continuous Cycling Peritoneal Dialysis using cycler machine usually during the night; with shorter dwell times than CAPD but more exchanges and commonly with a long dwell, or even an exchange, during the day
• CCPD with abdomen dry during the day may be called intermittent PD (IPD) or nocturnal intermittent PD (NIPD) performed as frequent, short cycles during the night with no day-time dwell
• TPD - tidal peritoneal dialysis (series of quick fills with incomplete drains, so that some residual volume [1/2 of usual dwell volume] remains in the peritoneal space; used infrequently as a peritoneal "conditioning" regimen)
Continuous flow
• CFPD - Continuous flow PD (requires double-lumen catheter or two separate catheters to support continuous flow of dialysate to increase efficiency; rarely used)

14.9.2 Peritoneal dialysis prescription

Adequate prescription of PD should provide adequate clearance, volume removal, and fit patient's lifestyle/schedule. Peritoneal dialysis prescription includes PD modality, number of exchanges, volume of exchange, and dialysate solution osmolarity ("strength" of PD dialysate to ultrafilter off fluid is usually determined by dextrose concentration, though icodextrin is available to enhance ultrafiltration over a longer dwell time.)

The choice of the modality is based on transport characteristics of the peritoneal membrane determined by the Peritoneal Equilibration Test (PET). Volume and number of exchanges is determined based on target clearance. The "strength" of solution is based on target ultrafiltration rate and also on peritoneal membrane transport characteristics (PET results).

14.9.3 PET interpretation and dialysis modality selection

Since the test is cumbersome and time and labor consuming, modifications have been proposed, eg, mini-PET or PET at home.

In brief: After morning drain, 2 liters of dialysate containing 2.5% dextrose (2,500 mg/dL) are infused and dwelled for 4 hours, samples of dialysate and serum are taken at time 0, 2 hours, and 4 hours. Dialysate (D) and plasma (P) creatinine and dialysate glucose are measured to calculate creatinine D/P ratio and glucose Dt/D0 ratio. The results can be plotted on a graph to assess the peritoneal transport characteristics of the patient as a high or rapid transporter, average transporter, or low or slow transporter. The 4-hour values are shown below.

Transport Type	D/P Creatinine 4h	D4hr/D0 Glucose	PD Modality Suggested by Transport Type
High	0.82–1.03	<0.26	CAPD or CCPD with rapid short exchanges is needed
High average	0.66–0.81	0.26–0.38	Standard CAPD or CCPD will be effective
Low average	0.5–0.64	0.38–0.49	If residual renal CrCl >2 ml/min: standard CAPD or CCPD will be effective. If residual renal CrCl <2 ml/min: high dose CAPD or CCPD with day dwell is needed
Low	0.34–0.49	>0.49	High-dose CAPD, consider HD

14.9.4 Peritoneal dialysis adequacy

Creatinine clearance >60 L per week per 1.73 m^2 body surface area (Calculate using serum and dialysate creatinine measurements from a 24-hr collection of dialysate).

Weekly Kt/Vurea >1.7-2.0 (either just dialysis clearance or a combination of dialysis clearance and residual kidney function). Calculate from website: http://www.kt-v.net/ using addition of residual renal function if urine output is >100 ml/day. To calculate weekly Kt/V for peritoneal dialysis:

K=clearance of urea (not creatinine) - measured by timed urine or dialysate collection
t = 10080 min (per week)
V = 0.6 (for males) or 0.5 (for females) x body weight in Kg

14.9.5 Complications of peritoneal dialysis

Causes of turbid PD fluid

- Infection
- RBC (hemorrhage, ovulation, menses)
- Severe constipation
- Fibrin or other proteins may cause incomplete drainage
- Lipids (chylous ascites)
- Prolonged dwell time
- Pancreatitis
- Dihydropyridine calcium channel blockers

Infectious complication of PD

PD peritonitis

Causes of PD Peritonitis
Primary
Caused by exogenous PD fluid contamination
Secondary
Secondary to intra-abdominal causes: Diverticulitis, appendicitis, cholecystitis, bowel necrosis or perforation to be suspected by • Symptoms of the intra-abdominal disease • Multiple/unusual enteric organisms • Stool in dialysate • Elevated amylase
Symptoms of PD Peritonitis
• Turbid PD fluid • Symptoms of peritoneal inflammation (abdominal pain, nausea, diarrhea or ileus) • Symptoms of infection (fever, chills)
Findings
• Peritoneal WBC >100/µL, >50% polymorphonuclear cells on differential for common bacterial pathogens (may have lymphocyte predominance for fungal or tuberculous peritonitis) • Positive PD fluid culture and/or gram stain

Severe Infection if	
• Symptoms > 24 hours • Severe pain • Vomiting • Fever > 101° • Hypotension or symptoms suggestive of sepsis • Patient unable to drain PD fluid	
Routes of Infection in PD Peritonitis	
Transluminal (touching or contaminating the catheter connection site)	30–40%
Periluminal (exit site or tunnel infection)	20–30%
Transmural (bowel seeding or perforation, diverticulitis, appendicitis, cholecystitis, severe constipation, colonoscopy)	25–35%
Hematogenous	5–10%
Ascending (female GU tract)	2–5%

Microorganisms in PD Peritonitis and Associated Mortality

Microorganism	Mortality rate
Staphylococcus epidermidis	<0.5%
Staphylococcus aureus	2.5%
Fungal	9.7%

Management of PD Peritonitis

• Send cell count and differential, culture and gram stain on initial drainage
• Start empiric antibiotics:
  - Cefazolin or cephalothin 15 mg/kg of body weight or 1 g/2-3 L bag QD (in the long dwell) and either
  - Ceftazidime or cefepime 10-15 mg/kg of body weight or 1 g/2-3 L bag QD (in the long dwell) or
  - Aminoglycoside (not recommended if residual urine output >100 ml/day): tobramycin or gentamicin, 0.6 mg/kg body weight in only 1 exchange per day or amikacin 2.0 mg/kg body weight, in only 1 exchange per day (or gentamicin 3 mg/kg IV) or
  - Oral quinolone (500 mg levofloxacin x 1, then 250 mg QD for 2 wks or ciprofloxacin 750 mg BID)
  - Refer patient to a hospital for symptoms of severe infection

Management of PD Peritonitis (cont.)

Culture in 24–48 hours

Culture positive:	Culture negative (20%)	Fungi (<2%)
Gram(+) (50%)	• No improvement: Repeat culture, continue antibiotics for 2 weeks	• Consider removing catheter which is often necessary
• Enterococci: Ampicillin 125 mg/L + aminoglycoside for 2 weeks in PD fluid	• Improvement: Discontinue aminoglycoside, continue cephalosporin for 2 weeks	• Fluconazole 150-200 mg every other day IP or amphotericin 25 mg/d IV and
• MSSA: Cephalosporin ± rifampin 600 mg PO for 3 weeks	• Often caused by coagulase (-) Staph	• Flucytosine load 2000 mg PO, maintenance 1000 mg PO for 4-6 weeks
• MRSA: Vancomycin 15-30 mg/kg in 1 bag per day, repeat every 3-7 days based on the level for 3 weeks	• Evaluate for other disease: TB, other mycobacterial or fungal peritonitis, eosinophilic peritonitis, intra-abdominal disease, renal cell or ovarian cancer, leukemia, lymphoma	• Change to Amphotericin if not better in 72 hours
• VRE: Remove catheter, Daptomycin 4-6mg/Kg/48h IV or linezolid 600mg/d PO or IV		
• Other: Stop aminoglycoside, continue cephalosporin for 2 weeks		
Gram(-) (15%)		
• Single G(-) non-Xanthomonas - adjust ABx to sensitivity *for 2 weeks*		
• Xanthomonas/Pseudomonas: Aminoglycoside + another anti-Pseudomonas ABx *for 3 weeks*		
• Multiple organisms/Anaerobes: Add Metronidazole 500 Q8h IV/PO for *3 weeks*, consider possible bowel perforation if not better in 72 h		

Indications for catheter removal

• Refractory/relapsing peritonitis
• Peritonitis associated with tunnel infection
• Unresponsive Pseudomonas or fungal peritonitis
• Fecal peritonitis or other significant intraabdominal pathology
• Mechanical failure of PD catheter

Acid-base and Electrolyte Disturbances in Peritoneal Dialysis

	Mechanism	Correction
Hypernatremia	Hypertonic dialysate ⇒ water shift into peritoneal space (removing water in excess of Na)	Water orally or D5W IV or lower glucose or Na level in dialysate
Hyponatremia	Low Na intake, excessive thirst, renal or stool losses, inadequate UF	Salt intake must be proportional to the volume loss induced by dialysis, increase hypertonic dialysate if water overload
Hyperkalemia	High K intake with low renal excretion, extracellular shift of K due to low insulin or drugs	Higher dialysis clearance, standard treatment of acute hyperkalemia
Hypokalemia	Excessive K^+ clearance by PD, occurs in 60% of ESRD patients on PD	10-30% of patients need K^+ supplement
Lactic acidosis	Conversion of lactate to bicarbonate can be affected in sepsis or by metformin	Replace lactate buffer with bicarbonate in dialysate

Hemoperitoneum

Causes of Hemoperitoneum

Benign causes	More serious causes
• Ovulation • Menstruation • Post-lithotripsy • Laparoscopic cholecystectomy • Shedding of ectopic endometrium	• Femoral hematoma leakage • Cyst rupture in PKD • Hematologic: Low platelets, coagulopathy • Adenocarcinoma of the colon • Ischemic bowel • Splenic rupture • Pancreatitis • Sclerosing peritonitis

Treatment
- Intraperitoneal heparin (does not change systemic coagulation, but prevents clotting of the catheter)
- If benign - observe
- If no obvious cause - investigate, e.g., PD fluid cytology, CT scan, etc.

Non-infectious complications of PD

Conditions	Diagnosis	Treatment
Hernia (↑ intraabdominal pressure)	Clinical examination or CT scan	Surgical repair, corsets, dialysis with lower intra-abdominal pressure (APD, eliminate daytime dwell or decrease volume)
Genital edema (< 10% CAPD Pts): Tracking of PD fluid to scrotum/labia	Clinical exam, decreased PD fluid effluent return, Ultra-sound/CT scan	Stop PD and use temporary HD, low volume APD at bed rest, further treatment depends on source of leak
Abdominal wall leak	Clinical exam, decreased PD fluid effluent return, Ultra-sound/CT scan	Stop PD and use temporary HD, low volume APD at bed rest, consider catheter replacement or injecting fibrin glue (1 ml of a solution of fibrinogen and thrombin)
Hydrothorax/Pleural effusion (incidence < 5%)	Dyspnea, no improvement with hypertonic exchange, decreased PD fluid effluent return, diagnostic CXR with pleural effusion, thoracentesis with pleural fluid analysis showing high glucose, scan with isotope in abdomen	Stop PD and use temporary HD, thoracentesis, low volume PD (after 2 wks of HD may return to PD), pleurodesis (fibrin glue, autologous blood, talc, tetracycline), surgical repair
Sclerosing encapsulating peritonitis	Recurrent abdominal pain with fills, repeated peritonitis predisposes to it, may cause bowel obstruction, or hemoperitoneum, decreased solute and water transport, characteristic appearance with CT	Careful attention to nutrition and bowel function, laparoscopy, surgical intervention, anti-inflammatory or immunosuppressive meds (controversial), tamoxifen

References and Suggested Reading

Dialysis Indications

Moss AH. Ethical principles and processes guiding dialysis decision-making. Clin J Am Soc Nephrol 2011;6(9):2313-2317.

Wright S, Klausner D, Baird B, et al. Timing of dialysis initiation and survival in ESRD. Clin J Am Soc Nephrol 2010;5(10):1828-1835.

Da Silva-Gane M, Wellsted D, Greenshields H, et al. Quality of life and survival in patients with advanced kidney failure managed conservatively or by dialysis. Clin J Am Soc Nephrol 2012;7(12):2002-2009.

Mehrotra R. Choice of dialysis modality. Kidney internat 2011;80(9):909-911.

Cooper BA, Branley P, Bulfone L, et al. A randomized, controlled trial of early versus late initiation of dialysis. N Engl J Med 2010;363(7):609-619.

do Nascimento GV, Gabriel DP, Abrao JM, Balbi AL. When is dialysis indicated in acute kidney injury? Ren Fail 2010;32(3):396-400.

Tolwani A. Continuous renal-replacement therapy for acute kidney injury. New Engl J Med 2012;367(26):2505-14.

Shiao CC, Wu VC, Li WY, et al. Late initiation of renal replacement therapy is associated with worse outcomes in acute kidney injury after major abdominal surgery. Crit Care. 2009;13(5):R171.

Vascular Access, Infection and Anticoagulation

DeSilva RN, Sandhu GS, Garg J, Goldfarb-Rumyantzev AS. Association between initial type of hemodialysis access used in the elderly and mortality. Hemodialysis International. 2012;16(2):233-41.

Allon M. Dialysis catheter-related bacteremia: treatment and prophylaxis. Am J Kidney Dis 2004;44(5):779-791.

Ramritu P, Halton K, Collignon P, et al. A systematic review comparing the relative effectiveness of antimicrobial-coated catheters in intensive care units. Am J Infect Control 2008;36(2):104-117.

Maaskant JM, De Boer JP, Dalesio O, et al. The effectiveness of chlorhexidine-silver sulfadiazine impregnated central venous catheters in patients receiving high-dose chemotherapy followed by peripheral stem cell transplantation. Eur J Cancer Care (Engl) 2009;18(5):477-482.

Babycos CR, Barrocas A, Webb WR. A prospective randomized trial comparing the silver-impregnated collagen cuff with the bedside tunneled subclavian catheter. JPEN J Parenter Enteral Nutr 1993;17(1):61-63.

James MT, Conley J, Tonelli M, et al for Alberta Kidney Disease Network. Meta-analysis: antibiotics for prophylaxis against hemodialysis catheter-related infections. Ann Intern Med 2008;148(8):596-605.

Rabindranath KS, Bansal T, Adams J, et al. Systematic review of antimicrobials for the prevention of haemodialysis catheter-related infections. Nephrol Dial Transplant 2009;24(12):3763-74.

Shaffer D. Catheter-related sepsis complicating long-term, tunnelled central venous dialysis catheters: management by guidewire exchange. Am J Kidney Dis 1995;25(4):593-596.

Beathard GA. Management of bacteremia associated with tunneled-cuffed hemodialysis catheters. J Am Soc Nephrol 1999;10(5):1045-1049.

Marr KA, Sexton DJ, Conlon PJ, et al. Catheter-related bacteremia and outcome of attempted catheter salvage in patients undergoing hemodialysis. Ann Intern Med 1997;127(4):275-280.

Launay-Vacher V, Izzedine H, Mercadal L, Deray G. Clinical review: use of vancomycin in haemodialysis patients. Crit Care 2002;6(4):313-316.

Daeihagh P, Jordan J, Chen J, Rocco M. Efficacy of tissue plasminogen activator administration on patency of hemodialysis access catheters. Am J Kidney Dis 2000;36(1):75-79.

Cronin RE, Reilly RF. Unfractionated heparin for hemodialysis: still the best option. Semin Dial 2010;23(5):510-515.

Swartz R, Pasko D, O'Toole J, Starmann B. Improving the delivery of continuous renal replacement therapy using regional citrate anticoagulation. Clin Nephrol 2004;61(2):134-143.

References and Suggested Reading (cont.)

Hemodialysis Adequacy

Eknoyan G, Beck GJ, Cheung AK, et al. Effect of dialysis dose and membrane flux in maintenance hemodialysis. N Engl J Med 2002;347(25):2010-2019.

Goldfarb-Rumyantzev AS, Schwenk MH, Liu S, et al. New empiric expressions to calculate single pool Kt/V and equilibriated Kt/V. ASAIO J 2002;48(5):570-576.

Hemodialysis Adequacy 2006 Work Group. Clinical practice guidelines for hemodialysis adequacy, update 2006. Am J Kidney Dis 2006; 48 Suppl 1:S2-90.

Daugirdas JT. Hemodialysis adequacy and biocompatibility. Seminars in dialysis. 2011; (5):508-9.

Bosch J, Beck W, Buck R, Shideman J. Polyflux ® Revaclear: The Next Generation in High-Flux Dialyzers. http://www.gambro.com/PageFiles/7915/2009%20Revaclear%20White%20Paper%20-%20306150163_B.pdf?epslanguage=en" Accessed Sep 12, 2012.

Ward RA, Ronco C. Dialyzer and machine technologies: application of recent advances to clinical practice. Blood Purif 2006;24(1):6-10

Peritoneal Dialysis

Liakopoulos V, Stefanidis I, Dombros NV. Peritoneal dialysis glossary 2009. Int Urol Nephrol 2010;42(2):417-423.

Twardowski ZJ. Peritoneal dialysis glossary III. Perit Dial Int 1990;10(2):173-175.

La Milia V, Di Filippo S, Crepaldi M, et al. Mini-peritoneal equilibration test: A simple and fast method to assess free water and small solute transport across the peritoneal membrane. Kidney Int 2005;68(2): 840-846.

Twardowski Z, Nolph K, Khanna R, al e. Peritoneal equilibration test. Perit Dial Bull 1987;7:138.

Peritoneal Dialysis Adequacy

Peritoneal Dialysis Adequacy 2006 Work Group. Clinical practice guidelines for peritoneal adequacy, update 2006. Am J Kidney Dis. 2006 Jul;48 Suppl 1:S91-7; also see S98-129 and S130-58.

Paniagua R, Amato D, Vonesh E, et al. Effects of increased peritoneal clearances on mortality rates in peritoneal dialysis: ADEMEX, a prospective, randomized, controlled trial. J Am Soc Nephrol 2002;13(5): 1307-1320.

Keane WF, Bailie GR, Boeschoten E, et al. Adult peritoneal dialysis-related peritonitis treatment recommendations: 2000 update. Perit Dial Int 2000;20(4):396-411.

PD Complications

Pérez Fontan M, Rodriguez-Carmona A, García-Naveiro R, et al. Peritonitis-related mortality in patients undergoing chronic peritoneal dialysis. Perit Dial Int. 2005;25(3):274-84

Piraino B, Bailie GR, Bernardini J, et al. for ISPD Ad Hoc Advisory Committee. Peritoneal dialysis-related infections recommendations: 2005 update. Perit Dial Int. 2005;25(2):107-31.

Yeung SM, Walker SE, Tailor SA, et al. Pharmacokinetics of oral ciprofloxacin in continuous cycling peritoneal dialysis. Perit Dial Int 2004;24(5):447-453.

Herbrig K, Pistrosch F, Gross P, Palm C. Resumption of peritoneal dialysis after transcutaneous treatment of a peritoneal leakage using fibrin glue. Nephrol Dial Transplant 2006;21(7):2037-2038.

References and Suggested Reading (cont.)

Kropp J, Sinsakul M, Butsch J, Rodby R. Laparoscopy in the early diagnosis and management of sclerosing encapsulating peritonitis. Semin Dial 2009;22(3):304-307.

Allaria PM, Giangrande A, Gandini E, Pisoni IB. Continuous ambulatory peritoneal dialysis and sclerosing encapsulating peritonitis: tamoxifen as a new therapeutic agent? J Nephrol 1999;12(6):395-397.

Uribarri J, Prabhakar S, Kahn T. Hyponatremia in peritoneal dialysis patients. Clin Nephrol 2004;61(1): 54-58.

Zanger R. Hyponatremia and hypokalemia in patients on peritoneal dialysis. Semin Dial 2010;23(6): 575-580.

Otte K, Gonzalez MT, Bajo MA, et al. Clinical experience with a new bicarbonate (25 mmol/L)/lactate (10 mmol/L) peritoneal dialysis solution. Perit Dial Int 2003;23(2):138-145.

Rodriguez-Carmona A, Pérez Fontán M, García López E, et al. Use of icodextrin during nocturnal auto-mated peritoneal dialysis allows sustained ultrafiltration while reducing the peritoneal glucose load: a randomized crossover study. Perit Dial Int 2007; 27(3):260-6.

15   Kidney Transplantation

Kidney transplantation represents a complex overlapping of immunology, nephrology, and surgery. In this chapter, we will describe the role of tissue typing and tissue compatibility in donor-recipient selection, immunosuppression, clinical aspects of kidney transplantation, its success rates and complications, including rejection and antirejection treatment.

At the end of the chapter, there is a theoretical description which provides several immunologic concepts important for understanding alloreactivity, the cells and molecules participating in the immune response, antigen recognition and rejection, and the effect of our immunosuppressive medications.

15.1   Tissue Typing & Compatibility

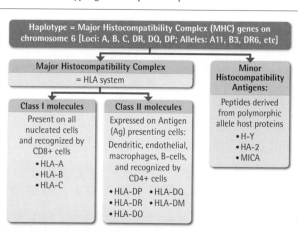

Haplotype = Major Histocompatibility Complex (MHC) genes on chromosome 6 [Loci: A, B, C, DR, DQ, DP; Alleles: A11, B3, DR6, etc]

Major Histocompatibility Complex
= HLA system

Minor Histocompatibility Antigens:
Peptides derived from polymorphic allele host proteins
• H-Y
• HA-2
• MICA

Class I molecules
Present on all nucleated cells and recognized by CD8+ cells
• HLA-A
• HLA-B
• HLA-C

Class II molecules
Expressed on Antigen (Ag) presenting cells:
Dendritic, endothelial, macrophages, B-cells, and recognized by CD4+ cells
• HLA-DP   • HLA-DQ
• HLA-DR   • HLA-DM
• HLA-DO

HLA -A, -B, -DR antigens are the most important in transplant rejection so, based on 2 alleles at each of these three loci, antigen matches can be from 0/6 to 6/6

Histocompatibility testing

- **Tissue typing**
  - Serological (identifying Ag on cell membranes: Reaction between cells of the subjects and antibodies to specific HLA antigens): Microlymphocytotoxicity test
  - Molecular techniques (DNA typing): PCR (DNA nomenclature: name has 4 digits, first 2 correlate with serologic name: A1, B3, etc; last 2 indicate allelic name)
- **HLA antibody (Ab) identification** (panel reactive antibodies - PRA) - Cytotoxic test, ELISA, flow cytometry
- **Crossmatching with T- and B- lymphocytes** (to predict hyperacute rejection): With B-cell - one is testing for class 1 antigens (A, B, C), presented only on B-cells and antigen presenting cells (APC) and is more important with T-cell testing discriminating class 1 and 2 (DR, DQ, DP) antigens; class 2 present on all nucleated cells
  - Microlymphocytotoxicity test with patient's serum and donor's lymphocytes (T & B) - screen for preformed Ab
  - Flow cytometry (flow cytometric crossmatch [FCXM] method): More sensitive, allows the detection of antibodies against T-lymphocytes (anti-HLA class I antibodies) and B-lymphocytes (anti-HLA class I and/or HLA class II antibodies)
  - Antiglobulin crossmatch

Lymphocytotoxicity test used in almost all of the above tests (complement-dependent cytotoxicity or CDC assay):
Ag + Ab + complement → lysis of lymphocytes (may be used to look for specific Ag or Ab)

15.2   Donor Selection & the Role of Tissue Matching

- **Blood type**: While there are some programs that transplant across incompatible ABO blood groups, typically it is required that donor and recipient would have the same or compatible blood type
- **HLA match**: Higher degree of HLA match is associated with proportionally increased long-term graft survival. Matching only for the alleles of HLA-A, -B, and -DR is considered for practical purposes
- **Preformed donor antibodies**: Presence of preformed antibodies against donor-specific HLA antigens is a barrier to transplantation and an important cause of allograft loss increasing the risk for early antibody-mediated rejection. Desensitization protocols can be used: Plasmapheresis, IV Ig, immunoabsorption, Rituximab

15.3 Factors Affecting Transplant Graft Outcome

15.3.1 Donor characteristics
• Live vs deceased donor
• Age
• BMI
• Race (worse outcome with Black or Hispanic donors)
• Gender (better with kidneys from males)
• Comorbidities
• Terminal creatinine level (for deceased donors)

15.3.2 Recipient characteristics
• Age, race (worse outcome in Black recipients), BMI, gender (better in males)
• First transplant (outcome of each consecutive transplant is generally worse)
• Renal replacement therapy (RRT) modality (PD or prior transplant are both better than HD)
• Timing of transplant - see charts below
• Duration of ESRD
• Cause of ESRD (eg, SLE is associated with inferior outcome)
• Presence of CVD
• Individual socio-economic factors (education level, type of insurance, alcohol use) and composite social adaptability index (higher index is associated with better outcome)

15.3.3 Other factors
• HLA match of donor and recipient
• Cold ischemia time of kidney
• Procedure (worse outcome with kidney-pancreas, en-bloc transplant)
• Higher transplant volume of transplant center
• State of the economy

15.4 Timing of Transplantation

First transplant	Re-transplantation
• Preemptive transplantation seems to be beneficial • However, being on dialysis for up to 6 months is associated with the same outcome as preemptive transplantation	• Unlike the first transplant, preemptive re-transplantation might be associated with a higher risk of graft loss by 36% • However, among those on dialysis in between transplants, longer time on dialysis is associated with higher risk

15.5 Preemptive Transplantation vs. Transplantation After Initial Period of Dialysis

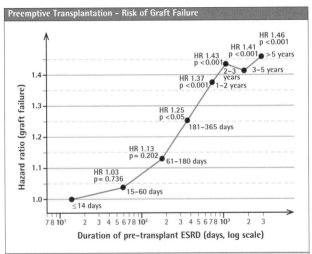

Goldfarb-Rumyantzev A, Hurdle JF, Scandling J, et al. Duration of end-stage renal disease and kidney transplant outcome. Nephrol Dial Transplant. 2005 Jan; 20(1):167-75. By permission of Oxford University Press and ERA-EDTA

Transplantation After Initial Period of Dialysis - Risk of Death

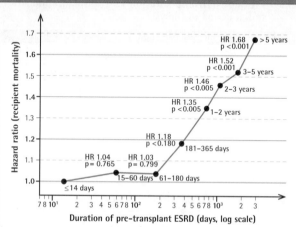

Goldfarb-Rumyantzev A, Hurdle JF, Scandling J, et al. Duration of end-stage renal disease and kidney transplant outcome. Nephrol Dial Transplant. 2005 Jan; 20(1):167-75. By permission of Oxford University Press and ERA-EDTA

15.6 Immunosuppression

15.6.1 Mechanism of action of immunosuppressive medications

The following diagram is a schematic representation of the mechanism of action of the most commonly used immunosuppressive medications (see immunologic pathways described at the end of this chapter).

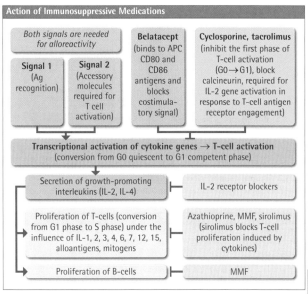

Action of Immunosuppressive Medications

Both signals are needed for alloreactivity

| **Signal 1** (Ag recognition) | **Signal 2** (Accessory molecules required for T cell activation) | **Belatacept** (binds to APC CD80 and CD86 antigens and blocks costimulatory signal) | **Cyclosporine, tacrolimus** (inhibit the first phase of T-cell activation (G0 → G1), block calcineurin, required for IL-2 gene activation in response to T-cell antigen receptor engagement) |

Transcriptional activation of cytokine genes → T-cell activation (conversion from G0 quiescent to G1 competent phase)

Secretion of growth-promoting interleukins (IL-2, IL-4)	IL-2 receptor blockers
Proliferation of T-cells (conversion from G1 phase to S phase) under the influence of IL-1, 2, 3, 4, 6, 7, 12, 15, alloantigens, mitogens	**Azathioprine, MMF, sirolimus** (sirolimus blocks T-cell proliferation induced by cytokines)
Proliferation of B-cells	MMF

The goal of immunosuppression therapy is suppressing the immune system to the point of avoiding rejection, but at the same time to minimize the potential side effects of excessive immune suppression.

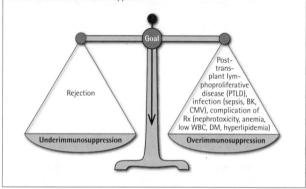

15.6.2 Immunosuppressive Medications

This table represents a summary of the mechanisms of action, doses, and side effects of the most commonly used immunosuppressive medications.

Cyclosporine (Neoral, Sandimmune)	
Mechanism	• Binds with cyclophyllin, this complex inhibits calcineurin $\Rightarrow$ $\downarrow$ expression of T-cell activation genes • Inhibits IL-2 driven proliferation of activated T cells (inhibits IL-2 message): Affects G0 to G1 cell cycle • Enhances the expression of TGF-β
Initial dose	• PO: 8–15 mg/kg/day, change in 2 mg/kg increments according to level • IV daily dose = 1/3 PO daily dose • Levels may be influenced by drugs affecting p-450 liver enzymes

Cyclosporine (Neoral, Sandimmune)	
Complications	• Nephrotoxicity (**Acute:** Reduction of renal blood flow b/o increased sympathetic tone and RA system; **chronic:** Interstitial fibrosis after 6-12 months of treatment b/o chronic ischemia and toxicity and enhanced apoptosis) • HTN • Hyperlipidemia • DM (less than tacrolimus) • CMV and other infections (as all other immunosuppressives) • ↓ T-cell proliferation • Tremors • Hirsutism • Hepatotoxicity • CNS toxicity • Gingival hypertrophy • Renal vascular damage • Malignancies

Tacrolimus (FK506, Prograf)	
Mechanism	• Similar to cyclosporine: Tacrolimus binds with FKBP12, this complex blocks calcineurin • Inhibits IL-2 (inhibits IL-2 message), -3, -4, TNF production • Affects G0 to G1 cell cycle
Initial dose	• 0.15-0.3 mg/kg/day
Complications	Similar to cyclosporine: • Nephrotoxicity (same as for cyclosporine) • Neurotoxicity (tremor, low seizure threshold, headaches, nightmares) • HTN • Hyperlipidemia (less than cyclosporine and sirolimus) • GI: Diarrhea, anorexia • Glucose intolerance/DM • CMV and other infections (as all other immunosuppressives) • Hyperkalemia • Malignancies

Sirolimus (Rapamycin)	
Mechanism	• Binds with FKBP12, interferes with TOR (Target of Rapamycin) and blocks T-cell activation, blocks IL-2 response • Affects G1 to S cell cycle
Initial dose	Start at 2 mg/day and follow levels
Complications	• Hypercholesterolemia, hypertriglyceridemia (treat with statins) • Stomatitis (dose reduction or transient DC) • Myelosuppression: Pancytopenia including thrombocytopenia (more common in combination with MMF, responds to dose reduction or transient DC) • HTN (treatment of choice: ACEI/ARB, but may worsen anemia) • Wound/incision complications, lymphocele (more common with high levels, in DM and obesity, responds to dose reduction or transient DC) • Pneumonitis (interstitial lung disease/BOOP/ pulmonary fibrosis: increased risk with higher level, may respond to dose reduction or DC) • May potentiate nephrotoxic effect of calcineurin inhibitors, increases MMF level (but not tacrolimus level) • CMV and other infections (as all other immunosuppressives) • Asthenia, headaches, epistaxis, diarrhea, arthralgias

Azathioprine (Imuran)	
Mechanism	• Inhibits purine nucleotide synthesis ⇒ inhibits gene replication & T-cell activation, suppresses myelocytes. Effectiveness is not blood level dependent
Initial dose	• Start 3–4 mg/kg/day, adjust the dose to WBC count • IV daily dose = 1/2 PO daily dose
Complications	• Bone marrow suppression/leukopenia • Hepatitis, cholestasis - occasionally

Mycophenolate mofetil (CellCept)	
Mechanism	• Active metabolite, mycophenolic acid (MPA) inhibits inosine monophosphate dehydrogenase (IMPDH), inhibits IL-2 production (inhibits IL-2 message) and response. • Inhibits de novo pathway of purine biosynthesis by blocking inosine monophosphate dehydrogenase activity. Blocks proliferation of T- and B-cells, Ab formation, generation of cytotoxic T-cells.

Initial dose	• 1000 mg PO twice a day (1500 mg twice a day when greater immunosuppression is desired)
Complications	• Gastrointestinal: dyspepsia, diarrhea, hepatic injury • Hematologic: leukopenia, anemia • CMV and other infections (as all other immunosuppressives)
Corticosteroids	
Mechanism	• Inhibit the expression of cytokine genes: IL-1, -2, -3, -6, TNF-α, γ-interferon • Nonspecific immunosuppresive effect
Initial dose	• Taper to 5 mg/day, or stop early if on early steroid withdrawal protocol
Complications	• Cataract, glaucoma • Hypertension, increased blood sugar levels • Osteoporosis, weight gain, water retention, puffy face, acne • Mood swings, irritability
Non - lymphocyte depleting antibodies – IL-2 inhibitors: Basiliximab (Simulect)	
Mechanism	• Monoclonal Ab's against IL-2 receptors. Used for induction therapy. For Pt's with high risk: retransplant, blacks, sensitized (PRA >30%), as induction in pancreas transplant
Initial dose	• Basiliximab 20 mg on day of surgery, again on POD#4
Complications	• Basiliximab: Nephrotoxicity
Lymphocyte depleting antibodies: Antithymocyte globulin equine (Atgam or ATG) or rabbit (Thymoglobulin or TMG)	
Mechanism	• Abs against CD3 reducing & blocking function of T lympho-cytes
Initial dose	• Dose may vary, eg, for induction with ATG 1.25mg/kg IV every other day for 3 doses
Complications	• Malignancies (PTLD)

Post-transplant Medications – 1

Typical initial post-transplant medications

Initial immunosuppressive regimen

- Calcineurin inhibitors (CNI) (tacrolimus or cyclosporine) **and**
- Antimetabolite (mycophenolate mofetil or azathioprine or sirolimus) **and**
- Prednisone (sometimes rapidly withdrawn)
- Sirolimus can be used in different combinations
- Induction with ATG or Basiliximab if: PRA >30%, blacks, kidney-pancreas transplant

Other

- Anti-HTN Rx
- Lipid-lowering medications if needed

Prophylactic medications

- Antiviral: CMV/herpes (valganciclovir, ganciclovir or acyclovir; dose based on serum creatinine) for 3 months
- Bacterial and PCP prophylaxis (Bactrim 1 single-strength tablet a day) for 6–12 months
- Fungal prophylaxis, e.g., oral candidiasis (fluconazole 50 mg once a day) for 1 month
- Steroid ulcer prophylaxis (H2-blockers)

Advantages of Ca-channel blockers in post-Tx patients for HTN

- Vasodilatory
- Stimulate natriuresis
- Protective effect on delayed graft fuction (DGF)
- Reduce hyperfiltration, renal hypertrophy, proximal tubular hypermetabolism, renal calcinosis
- Inhibition of cyclosporine-induced platelet aggregation and release of thromboxane
- <u>IMPORTANT:</u> Non-dihydropyridine Ca-channel blockers (e.g., verapamil, diltiazem) increase calcineurin inhibitor levels.

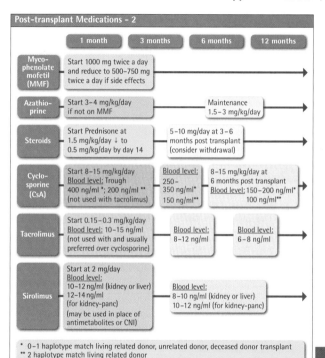

Post-transplant Medications – 2

	1 month	3 months	6 months	12 months
Myco-phenolate mofetil (MMF)	Start 1000 mg twice a day and reduce to 500–750 mg twice a day if side effects			
Azathio-prine	Start 3–4 mg/kg/day if not on MMF		Maintenance 1.5–3 mg/kg/day	
Steroids	Start Prednisone at 1.5 mg/kg/day ↓ to 0.5 mg/kg/day by day 14	5–10 mg/day at 3–6 months post transplant (consider withdrawal)		
Cyclo-sporine (CsA)	Start 8–15 mg/kg/day Blood level: Trough 400 ng/ml *: 200 ng/ml ** (not used with tacrolimus)	Blood level: 250–350 ng/ml* 150 ng/ml**	8–15 mg/kg/day at 6 months post transplant Blood level: 150–200 ng/ml* 100 ng/ml**	
Tacrolimus	Start 0.15–0.3 mg/kg/day Blood level: 10–15 ng/ml (not used with and usually preferred over cyclosporine)	Blood level: 8–12 ng/ml	Blood level: 6–8 ng/ml	
Sirolimus	Start at 2 mg/day Blood level: 10–12 ng/ml (kidney or liver) 12–14 ng/ml (for kidney-panc) (may be used in place of antimetabolites or CNI)	Blood level: 8–10 ng/ml (kidney or liver) 10–12 ng/ml (for kidney-panc)		

* 0–1 haplotype match living related donor, unrelated donor, deceased donor transplant
** 2 haplotype match living related donor

Change from oral to IV administration:
Tacrolimus 1/5 of the PO dose, Cyclosporine – 1/3 of the PO dose
MMF – the same dose, Azathioprine – 1/2 of the PO dose

15.6.3 Complications of maintenance immunosuppressive medications

	CsA	Tacro	MMF	Sirolimus
HTN	+++	++	-	-
Hyperlipid-emia	++	+	-	+++
Diabetes	+	+++	-	-
Nephrotoxic-ity	+++	+++	-	Associated with proteinuria and enhances toxicity of CsA and tacro
Diarrhea	+	++	+++	++ in combination with MMF
Anemia, leukopenia	-	-	++	++ especially in combination with MMF

15.6.4 Why convert from CNI (tacrolimus/cyclosporine) to sirolimus

- It inhibits growth factor-mediated proliferation of cells involved in chronic allograft nephropathy (CAN) pathogenesis
- It reduces the degree of vascular intimal thickening
- It helps to avoid underimmunosuppression
- It may be less nephrotoxic over time (creatinine preserved but can cause proteinuria) but has as many or more side effects as low dose CNI

Indications

- Nephrotoxicity of CNI (acute and chronic)
- Post-transplant diabetes
- Thrombotic microangiopathy (HUS)
- Poor initial graft function/extended criteria donor (old, HTN, DM/DGF/ischemic damaged kidneys/anatomic or surgical damage
- Side effects of CNI (hirsutism, gingival hyperplasia, neurotoxicity)
- Renal dysfunction in non-renal transplant patients
- Others: Polyoma, PTLD, etc
- Kaposi's sarcoma-treatable with sirolimus

Conversion protocol

Abrupt conversion (in ATN, diabetes, HUS)
- Stop CNI, after 24 h start sirolimus at loading dose 10 mg QD x2, then 5 mg QD
- Obtain blood level after 3rd dose and weekly
- Can decrease MMF if leukopenia

CNI overlap (in chronic allograft nephropathy)
- Decrease CNI by ½, start sirolimus at 5 mg/d
- Obtain blood level after 3rd dose and weekly
- Discontinue CNI when either sirolimus is therapeutic (8-12 ng/ml) or taper over 2-4 wks

Wait 24 before starting sirolimus for CsA/tac levels >250 or 14

May reduce MMF as levels are higher in combination with sirolimus

Medications Increasing CNI Level	Medications Decreasing CNI Level
• Ca-blockers, nondihydropyridines (eg, verapamil, diltiazem, nicardipine) • Antifungals (ketoconazole, fluconazole, itraconazole) • Antibiotics: Erythromycin & other macrolides • Histamine blockers (cimetidine) • Proton pump inhibitors (omeprazole) • Hormones (corticosteroids, oral contraceptives) • Grapefruit or grapefruit juice • Antiretroviral medications	• Anti-TB Rx (rifampin, INH) • Anticonvulsants (barbiturates, phenytoin, carbamazepine) • Antibiotics (nafcillin, IV trimethoprim, IV sulfa, imipenem, cephalosporins)

15.7 Early Kidney Transplant Complications & Allograft Dysfunction

15.7.1 Early complications of transplantation

- Mechanical
  - Leak (bleeding, lymphocele, urine leak)
  - Ureteral obstruction
  - Vascular thrombosis of artery or vein
- Medical
  - Delayed graft function
  - Rejection (accelerated acute/vascular rejection - no uptake on radioisotope scan; early cell mediated rejection - decreased radioisotope uptake)
  - Infection
  - Drug toxicity (cyclosporine/tacrolimus toxicity, associated thrombotic microangiopathy with HUS)
  - Volume depletion
  - De novo/recurrent renal disease
  - Other: ATN, prerenal failure, intrarenal conditions not specific for transplant kidney

Post-op Oliguria Management Algorithm

Post-op Oliguria Management

Irrigate bladder catheter

Check tacrolimus/cyclosporine level

Evaluate volume status (administer fluids or diuretics)

Ultrasound + doppler ± renal radioisotope scan

Kidney transplant biopsy

15.8   Delayed or Slow Graft Function

15.8.1 Delayed graft function (DGF)
- Requirement for dialysis in the first week
- Causes: ATN, antibody-mediated rejection, cortical necrosis/infarction, endothelial damage, thrombotic microangiopathy, drug-induced interstitial nephritis, fulminant disease recurrence.
- DGF of more than 6 days strongly decreases long-term survival of transplanted kidneys

15.8.2 Slow graft function
Serum creatinine >3 mg/dL without dialysis in the first week

15.9   Causes of Proteinuria in Post-transplant Patients

- De novo or recurrent GN
- Chronic rejection (most common)
- Cyclosporine or tacrolimus toxicity
- Sirolimus use has been associated with proteinuria
- Reflux nephropathy
- Renal vein thrombosis

15.10   Renal Transplant Rejection

15.10.1 Acute rejection
Acute rejection is one of the common early complications of renal transplant. Chronic rejection, while indicated in the following diagram for completeness, will be discussed in more details below.

Rejection Process

Hyperacute rejection minutes to hours	Acute rejection 5 days–3 months	Accelerated rejection 2–4 days	Chronic rejection Starting at few weeks
Preformed antibodies	Humoral or cellular immunity	Humoral or cellular immunity	Immune and nonimmune injuries
Microvascular thrombosis and cortical necrosis. This form of rejection is rarely seen in the modern practice of transplantation	Tubulointerstitial mononuclear cell infiltration, invasion of the tubular basement membrane and endovasculitis	Microvascular thrombosis and cortical necrosis	Thickening and reduplication of the GBM (resembling MPGN), tubular atrophy, interstitial fibrosis, vascular lumen obliteration, glomerular sclerosis

5–10% humoral mediated	90% cell mediated
Ab against donor's endothelial cell Ag – activate complement – vascular injury; characterized by ATN-like picture, positive staining for C4d in peritubular capillaries	CD4+, CD8+ cells – secrete effector molecules (granzymes, perforins) – causing cellular apoptosis

Treatment	Treatment
• Plasmapheresis • IV immunoglobulins • Bortezomib and eculizumab	• Pulse dose steroids • Methylprednisolone 5 mg/Kg/d (maximum and commonly given dose 500 mg/d) IV for 3 consecutive days then oral prednisone daily

If there is a partial response:	If there is no response (steroid-resistant rejection) or more aggressive rejection:
Repeat steroid pulse therapy	Anti-T-cell antibodies: Anti-thymocyte globulin (ATG); or monoclonal anti-lymphocyte antibodies

15.10.2 Banff ('97 classification and '07 update) of acute renal allograft rejection

1. Normal
2. Antibody-mediated changes
    - C4d deposition without morphologic evidence of active rejection
    - Acute antibody-mediated rejection
    - Chronic active antibody-mediated rejection
3. Borderline changes ('suspicious' for acute T-cell-mediated rejection)
4. T-cell mediated rejection

Acute:
    - IA. Cases with significant interstitial infiltration (>25% of parenchyma affected, i2 or i3) and foci of moderate tubulitis (t2)
    - IB. Cases with significant interstitial infiltration (>25% of parenchyma affected, i2 or i3) and foci of severe tubulitis (t3)
    - IIA. Cases with mild-to-moderate intimal arteritis (v1)
    - IIB. Cases with severe intimal arteritis comprising >25% of the luminal area (v2)
    - III. Cases with 'transmural' arteritis and/or arterial fibrinoid change and necrosis of medial smooth muscle cells with accompanying lymphocytic inflammation (v3)

Chronic active T-cell-mediated rejection
5. Interstitial fibrosis and tubular atrophy, no evidence of any specific etiology
    - I. Mild interstitial fibrosis and tubular atrophy (<25% of cortical area)
    - II. Moderate interstitial fibrosis and tubular atrophy (26-50% of cortical area)
    - III. Severe interstitial fibrosis and tubular atrophy/ loss (>50% of cortical area)
6. Other: Changes not considered to be due to rejection-acute and/or chronic

15.11 Late Complications of Renal Transplant

15.11.1 Differential diagnosis of late allograft dysfunction

Mechanical

- Urine leak
- Ureteral obstruction
- Renal artery stenosis
- Vascular thrombosis

Acute medical issues

- Rejection (acute or chronic)
- Drug toxicity (cyclosporine/tacrolimus toxicity or other drug toxicities)
- Volume depletion
- Infection
- Other: ATN, prerenal, intrarenal conditions not specific for transplant kidney

Chronic medical issues: Long-term allograft failure

- Chronic allograft nephropathy
- Input factors (preexisting conditions in donor kidney, transplant process: ischemia, reperfusion injury)
- Immune factors (histocompatibility, presensitization, host responsiveness, acute rejection, alloantibody, "subclinical rejection")
- Load stresses (HTN, donor-recipient size disparity [mismatch of kidney size], gender, proteinuria, hyperlipidemia, drug toxicities, infectious agents - CMV, BK virus)
- De novo/recurrent renal disease

15.11.2 Five entities that describe the status of a renal allograft

- **Rejection:** Graft injury secondary to T-cell mediated rejection (tubulitis, endothelialitis, interstitial infiltrates) or alloantibody-mediated rejection.
- **Allograft nephropathy:** Tubular atrophy, interstitial fibrosis, fibrous intimal thickening of the arteries
- **Transplant glomerulopathy**
- **Specific diseases:** recurrent or de novo renal disease, BK nephropathy, HUS, calcineurin inhibitor toxicity as a primary disease, diabetic nephropathy, hypertensive renal disease)
- **Accelerating processes:** HTN causing acceleration of other diseases, calcineurin inhibitor causing acceleration of other diseases, diabetes, proteinuria, lipid abnormalities

15.11.3 Chronic allograft nephropathy (CAN)

Chronic allograft nephropathy is defined as a gradual progressive decline in renal function usually associated with proteinuria and HTN leading to graft failure. It is caused by immunologic and nonimmunologic factors.

CAN: Development & Progression Mechanism

Mechanism of development and progression of chronic allograft nephropathy

Injury caused by immunologic (chronic rejection) and nonimmunologic (drug toxicity, HTN, recurrent disease) factors

Tissue response to injury

Tissue invading inflammatory cells and activated graft parenchymal cells secrete inflammatory mediators:
- Proinflammatory cytokines: IL-1-beta, TNF-alpha
- Enzymes
- Growth factors: transforming growth factor-beta, platelet-derived growth factor
- Angiotensin-2
- Endothelin
- Plasminogen activator inhibitor type 1

Additional factors
- Increased glomerular blood flow and pressure
- Increased glomerular permeability characteristics
- Glomerular hypertrophy
- Endothelin
- Lipoprotein disorders secondary to uremia and proteinuria

Chronic allograft dysfunction diagnosis
- Progressive allograft dysfunction – biopsy unavailable or uninformative
- Chronic/fibrosing allograft rejection (biopsy diagnosis)
  - Active (evidence of immunological activity: active infiltrates, C4d staining)
  - Inactive – characteristic late sclerotic lesions – arterial, capillary – without activity
- Specific other disease (biopsy diagnosis): e.g. calcineurin toxicity, chronic BK virus infection
- Chronic allograft nephropathy (biopsy diagnosis): fibrosing lesions with no etiologically specific lesions

CAN: Pathology (typically tubular atrophy, interstitial fibrosis, intimal vascular thickening)
Light microscopy

• Glomerular lesions and sclerosis
  - Wrinkling and collapse of the glomerular tuft
  - Glomerular hypertrophy
  - Mesangial matrix expansion
  - Thickening of the GBM
  - Focal glomerulosclerosis
  - Chronic transplant glomerulopathy (may be a form of chronic rejection): Double contours of the basement membrane, mesangiolysis, progressive sclerosing changes
• Tubulo-interstitial and vascular lesions
  - Atherosclerosis/hyperplastic vasculopathy: concentric fibrous intimal thickening (migration of fibroblasts into the intima -> local proliferation and deposition of extracellular matrix proteins) often with vessel wall infiltration with macrophages, lymphocytes, foam cells; thickening of the internal elastic lamina
  - Multilayering of peritubular capillaries
  - Interstitial fibrosis and tubular atrophy and cell drop out

Immunofluorescence
Nondiagnostic pattern of Ig deposition (linear IgG deposition along GBM, granular deposits of IgA, IgG in peripheral capillary loops)
Electron microscopy
Circumferential multilamination of the peritubular capillary basement membranes

15.11.4 Specific features of chronic rejection

Immune/inflammatory damage to the allograft; one of the causes of chronic allograft nephropathy:

• Intimal proliferation/thickening, with intimal lymphocytes, and splintering and disruption of the elastic lamina with formation of neo-media and neo-intima
• Duplication of basement membrane (chronic allograft glomerulopathy)
• Duplication of capillary lamina densa in peritubular capillaries
• Peritubular capillary staining for C4d in frozen tissue
• Overexpression of VCAM-1 on peritubular capillaries

15.12 Risk of Recurrent Disease in Transplanted Kidney

Most diseases affecting the native kidney may recur in the kidney transplant with the notable exception of a few, eg, polycystic kidney disease, hereditary nephritis or Alport's syndrome.

Risk of Recurrence (%)	Graft Loss from Recurrence (%)	Predictors of Recurrence	Treatment
Focal segmental glomerular sclerosis			
20-50%	13-20%	Younger age, rapid progression of original disease with development of end-stage renal failure within 3 years, mesangial hypercellularity of native kidney, Caucasian race, history of previous graft failure due to recurrence	Plasma exchange, steroids, ACEI, possibly rituximab, changing from sirolimus back to CNI. Preemptive perioperative plasma exchange in those with high risk.
Membranous glomerulopathy			
10-30%	10-15%	Seropositivity for Anti-PLA2 receptor antibodies may offer future clinical test. Initial concerns with regard to the risk of recurrence with living related donors, presence of HLA-DR3 in the recipient, and the aggressiveness of native disease have not been substantiated	No role for additional immunosuppression, Rituximab (small case series)
Membranoproliferative glomerulonephritis, Type I			
20-30%	15% (in a second graft 80%)	HLA-B8 DR3, living related donors and previous graft loss from recurrence	ASA, dipyridamole

Risk of Recurrence (%)	Graft Loss from Recurrence (%)	Predictors of Recurrence	Treatment
Membranoproliferative glomerulonephritis, Type II			
80–100%	15–30%	Male gender, RPGN of original disease, nephrotic syndrome	Plasma exchange
IgA nephropathy			
15–60% (risk is increased 20–100% in second transplant)	1–10%	No single parameter including age, gender, race, HLA (although B35 and DR4 were suggested), pre-transplant course or biochemical characteristic of serum IgA can predict recurrence	In crescentic glomerulopathy: Plasma exchange, cytotoxics; otherwise no effective therapy except for ACEI/ARB
Henoch-Schönlein purpura			
30–75%	20–40%	–	Plasma exchange, possibly steroids
ANCA-associated glomerulonephritis/vasculitis			
17%	6–8%	–	It is advisable to defer kidney transplantation until the disease is inactive. Patients with renal relapses - cyclophosphamide. Patients with cellular crescents and high ANCA titer - cyclophosphamide + plasma exchange ± IV Ig
Anti-GBM nephritis			
Up to 50% if antibodies were still present	Rare	Positive anti-GBM antibodies	Pulse steroids, plasma exchange, cyclophosphamide, Ab immunoadsorption

Risk of Recurrence (%)	Graft Loss from Recurrence (%)	Predictors of Recurrence	Treatment
Hemolytic uremic syndrome			
13-25%	40-50%	-	Plasma exchange, possibly steroids, switch from CNI to alternate immuno-suppression
Lupus nephritis			
Histological recurrence up to 30%, but clinically significant recurrent disease occurs in only 2-9%	2-4%	-	Postpone renal transplantation until the disease become quiescent for at least 6-9 months. MMF for recurrence.
Granulomatosis with polyangiitis (Wegener's)			
Up to 70%	-	-	Cyclophosphamide ± plasma exchange
Alport's syndrome, hereditary nephritis			
<10% de novo "anti-GBM" RPGN	100%	-	-
Diabetes mellitus			
Histological features recur in most if not all patients	-	-	Same as for diabetic nephropathy

Causes of Graft Failure During 10 Years of Follow-up	
Chronic rejection/CAN	26-40%
Death with graft functioning	30-53%
Recurrent renal disease	3-6%
Acute rejection	0.6-7.5%
De novo renal disease	0.2-1%
Noncompliance with immunosuppressives	2-10%
Other	3-10%

15.13 Transplant Outcome (2011 data)

15.13.1 Survival in deceased donor transplant

	1 year	3 years	5 years	10 years
Graft survival	95.2%	90.6%	84%	70.4%
Patient survival	96.4%	92.4%	86.9%	73.6%

15.13.2 Survival in living donor transplant

	1 year	3 years	5 years	10 years
Graft survival	98.1%	94.9%	90.6%	77.3%
Patient survival	98.7%	96.4%	93.4%	83%

Data from Scientific Registry of Transplant Recipients (SRTR) The 2011 Annual Data Report;
http://srtr.transplant.hrsa.gov/annual_reports/2011/default.aspx

Kidney transplants showed improved survival in recipients whose native kidney disease was caused by the following etiologies (in order): HTN > DM > GN > PKD (with significant differences even when adjusted for co-factors).

15.14 Major Causes of Transplant Recipient Mortality

- Cardiovascular Disease
- Malignancy (see below)
- Infection (higher risk in those with diabetes, poor renal function, increased immunosuppression, leukopenia, seronegativity for CMV, splenectomy, and malnutrition)
- Liver Disease (viral hepatitis or related to medication toxicity)

15.15 Major Causes of Post-transplant Morbidity

- Hypertension
- Hyperlipidemia
- Posttransplant diabetes mellitus
- Neoplasms (see below)
- Electrolyte disturbances: Hyperkalemia, hypomagnesemia, hypophosphatemia
- Musculoskeletal disorders
- Erythocytosis (can usually be controlled with ACEI Rx)
- GI problems
- Ocular disease
- Nonmalignant skin disease (basal cell epitheliomas very commonly)
- Psychiatric disease
- Allograft failure

15.16 Malignancies

By 20 years post-transplant:
- Nearly 50% of recipients had ≥1 skin cancer
- Over 10% of recipients had a non-skin, non-PTLD (post-transplant lymphoprolif-erative disease) malignancy
- Over 2% of recipients developed PTLD

Most common post-transplant malignancies
- Squamous cell carcinomas of the skin
- Non-Hodgkin's lymphomas
- In situ carcinomas of the uterine cervix, vulva, and perineum
- Renal carcinomas
- Kaposi's sarcoma (sirolimus is effective Rx)
- Other carcinomas: 1.5-fold increased risk of developing cancers seen in the gen-eral population (eg, carcinomas of the lung and colon)

Note: Those who had cancer before Tx; are over age 55 years; have had intensive immunosuppressive therapy or many years of immunosuppressive therapy are at greater risk

Risk Factors for Malignancies in Transplant Recipients	
Transplant-specific	The degree of immunosuppression • Antibody induction therapy • Exposure: Dose, duration, type and number of medications Oncogenic viruses (see below)
	Association between viruses and specific malignancies • EBV: Post-transplant lymphoproliferative disease (PTLD). Risk is increased with EBV positive donor transplant in EBV negative recipient • Human herpes virus 8: Kaposi's sarcoma, PTLD • HPV: Cervical cancer, penile cancer, vulvar cancer • HPV 58: Bowen's disease • HPV 8, 19: Non-melanoma skin cancer • HPV 16, 20: Skin and tonsillar cancer • Hepatitis B and C viruses: Hepatocellular carcinoma
Conventional risk factors	• Smoking • Sun exposure • Analgesic abuse • History of previous malignancy • Age • Genetic predisposition

15.17 Post-transplant Infectious Complications and Prophylaxis

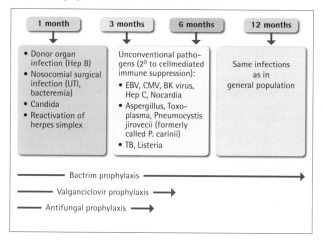

BK Virus

Diagnosis
- Plasma and urine: PCR, viral DNA, immunofixation, hemagglutinin inhibition
- Kidney Biopsy: signs of tubular injury, presence of intranuclear viral inclusions, immunohistochemistry to demonstrate infected tubular epithelial cells

Treatment
- Reduce or stop immunosuppression: Decrease MMF dose by 50%
- Substitute leflunomide for tacrolimus
- Cidofovir 0.5 mg/kg, or if impaired renal function 0.25-0.3 mg/kg.
- Follow PCR titers

15.18 Immunosuppression Withdrawal After Graft Failure

As it has been demonstrated that it is of potential benefit to go on dialysis in between transplants for those with repeat transplants, one of the potential mechanisms may be the withdrawal of immunosuppressive therapy. However, there are risks associated with immunosuppression withdrawal.

15.18.1 Complications of immunosuppression withdrawal
- Acute rejection, possibly requiring transplant nephrectomy (even after allograft failure)
- Secondary adrenal insufficiency after withdrawing prednisone
- Loss of residual renal function supported by allograft
- Sensitization in those who are candidates for another transplantation; transplant nephrectomy might limit sensitization

15.18.2 Strategies for immunosuppression withdrawal
- Early allograft failure (ie, less than one year after surgery): Immediate withdrawal of immunosuppression combined with preemptive nephrectomy may be advisable.
- Later allograft failure: Immediately withdraw cyclosporine or tacrolimus and azathioprine or mycophenolate mofetil; subsequently taper prednisone by 1 mg/month until the prednisone is discontinued, carefully watching for symptoms of adrenal insufficiency.
- Those who develop symptoms of allograft rejection with withdrawal can be treated as for acute rejection (3 days of pulse doses of Solu-Medrol), followed by tapering doses of oral prednisone then transplant nephrectomy may be advisable if long-term steroid is necessary

15.19 Transplant Patient Management

- General well-being, exercise, nutrition, appetite, weight, etc
- Kidney allograft function
- Immunosuppression: regimen, drug levels, side effects (e.g., tremor, osteoporosis, DM), taper prednisone, etc.
- Infection prophylaxis: symptoms of infection, medication adjustment of immunosuppressives and discontinuation, timing of antimicrobial prophylaxis
- HTN control
- DM or other primary disease status and control
- Anemia or post-transplant erythrocytosis management
- Cholesterol levels
- CKD management, if transplant is failing
- Primary care: bone disease, vaccinations (pneumococcus, 2-3yrs; flu,1yr), stool for occult blood (yearly)
  - CAD prophylaxis
  - Cancer screening and prophylaxis: Particularly with long-term or intense immunosuppression - sunscreen & skin exam (yearly), mammography (yearly), pap smears (2-3 years), colonoscopy (5yrs), PSA & CXR (uncertain data)

15.20 Elements of Hematopoiesis & Immunology
15.20.1 Types and origin of cells participating in immune response

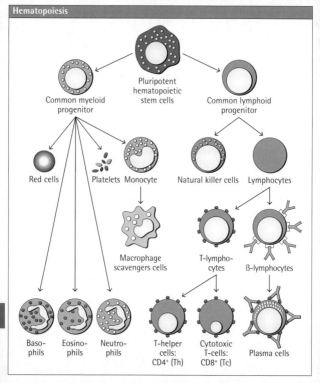

Hematopoiesis

Pluripotent hematopoietic stem cells

Common myeloid progenitor

Common lymphoid progenitor

Red cells

Platelets

Monocyte

Natural killer cells

Lymphocytes

Macrophage scavengers cells

T-lympho-cytes

ß-lymphocytes

Baso-phils

Eosino-phils

Neutro-phils

T-helper cells: CD4+ (Th)

Cytotoxic T-cells: CD8+ (Tc)

Plasma cells

15.20.2 Lymphocytes and their role in immune response

	Function	Receptors expressed
Natural killer cells	Lysis of virally infected cells and tumor cells	CD16, CD56, but not CD3
Helper T cells (Th)	Release cytokines and growth factors that regulate other immune cells	TCRαβ, CD3 and CD4
Cytotoxic T cells (Tc)	Lysis of virally infected cells, tumor cells and allografts	TCRαβ, CD3 and CD8
γ δ T cells	Immunoregulation and cytotoxicity	TCRγ δ and CD3
B cells	Secretion of antibodies	MHC class II, CD19, CD20 and CD21

15.20.3 The role of Th cells

T-helper (Th) lymphocytes consist of Th1 and Th2 subsets. Th1 cells are effectors of cell-mediated immunity and secrete interferon-gamma (IFN-gamma) along with multiple other cytokines. IFN-gamma in combination with IL-12 recruits new Th1 cells in cooperation with interleukin-12 produced by monocytes. IFN-gamma also inhibits differentiation of Th cells into Th2. Th2 cells, on the other hand, act more as a suppressors of immune response; they produce IL-4 and IL-10 along with other cytokines, which inhibit IFN-gamma secretion and cell immunity. In addition to Th1 and Th2, there are other Th cell types: Th3, Th17 (produce IL-17, important in auto-immune disease), ThFH.

We will now discuss the role of Th cells in regulating immune response. After the Th cell has been activated by the antigen-presenting cell (APC), it undergoes the process of differentiation into one of the Th subtypes and secretes multiple cytokines, involved in a complex process of regulation of the immune response as depicted in the following figure.

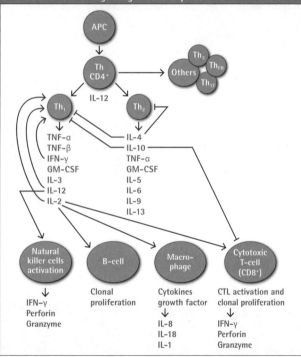

The Role of Th Cells in Regulating Immune Response

15.20.4 Th-cell activation

As indicated above, activated Th cells undergo the process of differentiation and secrete regulatory cytokines. The process of activating the Th cell is a function of the APC in which two signals are necessary to activate the Th cell as indicated in the following figure.

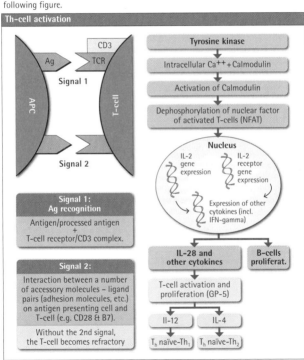

Th-cell activation

Signal 1: Ag recognition

Antigen/processed antigen + T-cell receptor/CD3 complex.

Signal 2:

Interaction between a number of accessory molecules – ligand pairs (adhesion molecules, etc.) on antigen presenting cell and T-cell (e.g. CD28 & B7).

Without the 2nd signal, the T-cell becomes refractory

15.20.5 Role of cytokines in developing tolerance

In addition to the immunologic reaction that leads to rejection of allogenic tissue, there are mechanisms of developing immunologic tolerance that prevents an allograft from being rejected. This process is also regulated by cytokines.

- IL-2 - essential for T-cell apoptosis
- IFN-gamma - down-regulates the proliferation of activated T-cells
- IL- 4 + IL-13 - converts T-cells into suppressor cells (Th1 $\rightarrow$ Th2 deviation)

15.20.6 Mechanism of allorecognition & adhesion

Allorecognition & Adhesion	
Direct allorecognition	• Donor APC - pepTide + recipient T-cells. Donor APC, still present in the allograft are necessary for this process. • This process has a role in acute rejection only, whereas after 2-3 months the graft is depleted of donor's leukocytes. • In addition to donor APC, donor endothelial cells can provide signal 1 (acting as an APC) and another cell (eg, macrophage/monocyte) can provide signal 2 to reactivate memory T-cells
Indirect allorecognition	• Recipient APC - donor peptide + recipient T-cells • This process has a greater role in chronic rejection. • Another mechanism involves endothelial cells: Endothelial cells promote stimulation and differentiation of APC into a dendritic cell. An APC comes to the site of inflammation or an allograft as a monocyte and emerges from the graft as a dendritic cell which reacts to an Ag from endothelial cells
Adhesion and recruitment	• Recruitment molecules on the surface of endothelial cells (eg, ICAM, selectines) $\rightarrow$ binding and activation of T-cells $\rightarrow$ increased expression of adhesion molecules

References and Suggested Reading

Donor-recipient selection, timing, and tissue typing

Sheldon S, Poulton K. HLA typing and its influence on organ transplantation. Methods Mol Biol. 2006;333:157–74.

Takemoto SK. HLA matching in the new millennium. Clin Transpl. 2003:387–403.

Delgado JC, Eckels DD. Positive B-cell only flow cytometric crossmatch: implications for renal transplantation. Exp Mol Pathol. 2008 Aug;85(1):59–63.

Goldfarb-Rumyantzev AS, Hurdle JF, Baird BC, et al. The role of pre-emptive re-transplant in graft and recipient outcome. Nephrol Dial Transplant. 2006 May;21(5):1355–64.

Kaneku H. Annual literature review of donor-specific HLA antibodies after organ transplantation. Clin Transpl. 2011:311–8.

Everly MJ. Donor-specific anti-HLA antibody monitoring and removal in solid organ transplant recipients. Clin Transpl. 2011:319–25.

Goldfarb-Rumyantzev AS, Hurdle JF, Scandling JD, et al.The role of pretransplantation renal replacement therapy modality in kidney allograft and recipient survival. Am J Kidney Dis. 2005 Sep;46(3):537–49.

Garg J, Karim M, Tang H, et al. Social adaptability index predicts kidney transplant outcome: a single-center retrospective analysis. Nephrol Dial Transplant. 2011 Mar;27(3):1239–45.

Gueye AS, Baird BC, Shihab F, et al. The role of the economic environment in kidney transplant outcomes. Clin Transplant. 2009 Sep–Oct;23(5):643–52.

Graft survival and loss

Scientific Registry of Transplant Recipients (SRTR). The 2011 Annual Data Report. Accessed Feb 26, 2013 at http://srtr.transplant.hrsa.gov/annual_reports/2011/default.aspx.

Nankivell BJ, Kuypers DR. Diagnosis and prevention of chronic kidney allograft loss. Lancet. 2011 Oct 15;378(9800):1428–37.

Racusen LC, Solez K, Colvin R. Fibrosis and atrophy in the renal allograft: interim report and new directions. Am J Transplant. 2002 Mar;2(3):203–6.

Colvin RB. Antibody-mediated renal allograft rejection: diagnosis and pathogenesis. J Am Soc Nephrol. 2007 Apr;18(4):1046–56.

Racusen LC, Haas M. Antibody-mediated rejection in renal allografts: lessons from pathology. Clin J Am Soc Nephrol. 2006 May;1(3):415–20.

Halloran PF. Call for revolution: a new approach to describing allograft deterioration. Am J Transplant. 2002 Mar;2(3):195–200.

Matas AJ, Gillingham KJ, Humar A, et al. 2202 kidney transplant recipients with 10 years of graft function: what happens next? Am J Transplant. 2008 Nov;8(11):2410–9.

Goldfarb-Rumyantzev AS, Scandling JD, Pappas L, et al. Prediction of 3-yr cadaveric graft survival based on pre-transplant variables in a large national dataset. Clin Transplant. 2003 Dec;17(6):485–97.

Goldfarb-Rumyantzev A, Hurdle JF, Scandling J, et al. Duration of end-stage renal disease and kidney transplant outcome. Nephrol Dial Transplant. 2005 Jan;20(1):167–75.

Tang H, Chelamcharla M, Baird BC, et al. Factors affecting kidney-transplant outcome in recipients with lupus nephritis. Clin Transplant. 2008 May–Jun;22(3):263–72

Chelamcharla M, Javaid B, Baird BC, Goldfarb-Rumyantzev AS. The outcome of renal transplantation among systemic lupus erythematosus patients. Nephrol Dial Transplant. 2007 Dec;22(12):3623–30.

Petersen E, Baird BC, Shihab F, et al. The impact of recipient history of cardiovascular disease on kidney transplant outcome. ASAIO J. 2007 Sep–Oct;53(5):601–8.

Goldfarb-Rumyantzev AS, Koford JK, Baird BC, et al. Role of socioeconomic status in kidney transplant outcome. Clin J Am Soc Nephrol. 2006 Mar;1(2):313–22.

References and Suggested Reading (cont.)

McGee J, Magnus JH, Islam TM, et al. Donor-recipient gender and size mismatch affects graft success after kidney transplantation. J Am Coll Surg 2010 May; 210:718-726.

Tan JC, Kim JP, Chertow GM, et al. Donor-recipient sex mismatch in kidney transplantation. Gend Med 2012 Oct; 9:335-347.

Vereerstraeten P, Wissing M, De Pauw L, et al. Male recipients of kidneys from female donors are at increased risk of graft loss from both rejection and technical failure. Clin Transplant 1999 Apr; 13:181-6.

Thomas MC, Mathew TH, Russ GR. Glycaemic control and graft loss following renal transplantation. Nephrol Dial Transplant. 2001 Oct;16(10):1978-82.

Krikov S, Khan A, Baird BC, et al. Predicting kidney transplant survival using tree-based modeling. ASAIO J. 2007 Sep-Oct;53(5):592-600.

Transplant kidney histopathology

Racusen LC, Solez K, Colvin RB, et al. The Banff 97 working classification of renal allograft pathology. Kidney Int. 1999 Feb;55(2):713-23.

Solez K, Colvin RB, Racusen LC, et al. Banff 07 classification of renal allograft pathology: updates and future directions. Am J Transplant. 2008 Apr;8(4):753-60.

Fletcher JT, Nankivell BJ, Alexander SI. Chronic allograft nephropathy. Pediatr Nephrol. 2009 Aug;24(8):1465-71.

Halloran PF, Melk A, Barth C. Rethinking chronic allograft nephropathy: the concept of accelerated senescence. J Am Soc Nephrol. 1999 Jan;10(1):167-81.

Complications of transplantation

Dall A, Hariharan S. BK virus nephritis after renal transplantation. Clin J Am Soc Nephrol. 2008 Mar;3 Suppl 2:S68-75.

Morath C, Mueller M, Goldschmidt H, et al. Malignancy in renal transplantation. J Am Soc Nephrol. 2004 Jun;15(6):1582-8.

Dantal J, Pohanka E. Malignancies in renal transplantation: an unmet medical need. Nephrol Dial Transplant. 2007 May;22 Suppl 1:i4-10.

Quinlan SC, Pfeiffer RM, Morton LM, Engels EA. Risk factors for early-onset and late-onset post-transplant lymphoproliferative disorder in kidney recipients in the United States. Am J Hematol. 2011 Feb;86(2):206-9.

Recurrent disease in the allograft

Golgert WA, Appel GB, Hariharan S. Recurrent glomerulonephritis after renal transplantation: an unsolved problem. Clin J Am Soc Nephrol. 2008 May;3(3):800-7.

Kotanko P, Pusey CD, Levy JB. Recurrent glomerulonephritis following renal transplantation. Transplantation. 1997 Apr 27;63(8):1045-52.

Hickson LJ, Gera M, Amer H, et al. Kidney transplantation for primary focal segmental glomerulosclerosis: outcomes and response to therapy for recurrence. Transplantation. 2009 Apr 27;87(8):1232-9.

Dabade TS, Grande JP, Norby SM, et al. Recurrent idiopathic membranous nephropathy after kidney transplantation: a surveillance biopsy study. Am J Transplant. 2008 Jun;8(6):1318-22.

El-Zoghby ZM, Grande JP, Fraile MG, et al. Recurrent idiopathic membranous nephropathy: early diagnosis by protocol biopsies and treatment with anti-CD20 monoclonal antibodies. Am J Transplant. 2009 Dec;9(12):2800-7.

References and Suggested Reading (cont.)

Choy BY, Chan TM, Lai KN. Recurrent glomerulonephritis after kidney transplantation. Am J Transplant. 2006 Nov;6(11):2535-42.

Lee J, Clayton F, Shihab F, Goldfarb-Rumyantzev A. Successful treatment of recurrent Henoch-Schönlein purpura in a renal allograft with plasmapheresis. Am J Transplant. 2008 Jan;8(1):228-31.

Beck LH Jr. Monoclonal anti-PLA2R and recurrent membranous nephropathy: Another piece of the puzzle. J Am Soc Nephrol 2012 Dec;23(12):1911-13.

Immunosuppression and transplant immunology

Saunders RN, Metcalfe MS, Nicholson ML. Rapamycin in transplantation: a review of the evidence. Kidney Int. 2001 Jan;59(1):3-16.

Gaston RS. Chronic calcineurin inhibitor nephrotoxicity: reflections on an evolving paradigm. Clin J Am Soc Nephrol. 2009 Dec;4(12):2029-34.

Bestard O, Campistol JM, Morales JM, et al. Advances in immunosuppression for kidney transplantation: new strategies for preserving kidney function and reducing cardiovascular risk. Nefrologia 2012 May 14;32(3):374-84.

Berrington JE, Barge D, Fenton AC, et al. Lymphocyte subsets in term and significantly preterm UK infants in the first year of life analysed by single platform flow cytometry. Clin Exp Immunol. 2005 May;140(2):289-92.

Chinen J, Buckley RH. Transplantation immunology: solid organ and bone marrow. J Allergy Clin Immunol. 2010 Feb;125(2 Suppl 2):S324-35.

Ekberg H, Bernasconi C, Tedesco-Silva H, et al. Calcineurin inhibitor minimization in the Symphony study: Observational results 3 years after transplantation. American Journal of Transplantation 2009; 9: 1876-1885.

Ekberg H, Bernasconi C, Nöldeke J, et al. Cyclosporine, tacrolimus and sirolimus retain their distinct toxicity profiles despite low doses in the Symphony study. Nephrol Dial Transplant. 2010 Jun; 25(6):2004-10.

16 Lab Values for Nephrology

16.1 Adrenocorticotropic Hormone (ACTH)

Adrenocorticotropic hormone (ACTH), plasma
Reference range
<120 pg/mL [SI units: <26 pmol/L]
Description
Polypeptide hormone of the anterior lobe of the pituitary gland (hypophysis) that stimulates growth of the adrenal cortex or secretion of its hormones. Indicator used in the differential diagnosis of hypercortisolism and adrenocortical insufficiency.
• **Increased:** Central Cushing syndrome - Pituitary ACTH secreting adenoma (usually microadenomas), hypothalamic hyperfunction (increased corticotropin-releasing hormone), ACTH therapy, Addison's disease • **Decreased:** Adrenal Cushing syndrome (adrenal adenoma, adrenal hyperplasia, adrenal carcinoma), iatrogenic hypercortisolism (long-term glucocorticoid therapy)

16.2 Albumin

Albumin, serum
Reference range
3.5 - 5.0 g/dL [SI units: 35-50 g/L]
Description
Albumin is a transport protein for small molecules, including bilirubin, calcium, progesterone and various medications. Its oncotic pressure serves to keep the fluid in the blood and avoid leaking out into the tissues. The test helps to assess protein absorption or malnutrition of body and to determine if patient has liver or kidney disease.
• **Increased:** Dehydration, shock • **Decreased:** Cystic fibrosis, proteinuric glomerular kidney disease, alcoholic cirrhosis, Hodgkin's disease, malnutrition, nephrotic syndrome, multiple myeloma, inflammatory bowel disease, leukemia, collagen-vascular diseases

16.3   Albumin/creatinine Ratio

Albumin/creatinine ratio, urine		
Reference range		
	On spot urine:	24 hour urine collection:
• Normal:	<30 mg/gm • <17 mg/gm (men) • <25 mg/gm (women)	• <30 mg/24h
• Microalbumin-uria:	30 -300 mg/gm (either sex) • 17 - 300 mg/gm (men) • 25 - 300 mg/gm (women)	• 30 - 300 mg/24h
• Macroalbumin-uria:	>300 mg/gm	• >300 mg/24h
Description		
It is used to measure albuminuria as a sign of kidney disease and in diabetes and hypertension which may lead to kidney disease or cardiovascular disease. **Microalbuminuria:** Chronic kidney disease, diabetes mellitus, congestive cardiac failure, acute or chronic obstructive airways disease, hypertension, malignancy		

16.4   Aldosterone

Aldosterone, plasma and urine
Reference range
• Plasma: 2-9 ng/dL [SI units 55-250 pmol/L] • Urine: 2-26 µg/day [SI units: 6-72 nmol/day]
Description
Adrenal glands release hormone aldosterone which maintains blood volume and pressure. Blood pressure increases, when aldosterone increases the reabsorption of sodium by the kidneys. It also causes renal excretion of potassium. Renin levels should usually be measured simultaneously to assess whether a high aldosterone is primary (low renin) or secondary (high renin). • **Increased:** Primary hyperaldosteronism, secondary hyperaldosteronism, very low-sodium diet • **Decreased:** Addison's disease, very high-sodium diet

16.5 Alkaline Phosphatase

Alkaline phosphatase, serum
Reference range
30-120 U/L [SI units: 0.5-2.0 µkat/L] (for adults)
Description
Group of enzymes that hydrolyze many orthophosphoric monoesters and that are present ubiquitously (liver, kidney, bones, intestine and placenta).

- **Increased:** Physiological-during growth, last trimester of pregnancy, rickets, osteomalacia, ulcerative colitis, bowel perforation, fatty liver, alcoholic hepatitis, hyperparathyroidism, hyperthyroidism
- **Decreased:** Vitamin D intoxication, pernicious anemia, hypothyroidism, celiac sprue, malnutrition, fibrate therapy

16.6 Amylase

Amylase
Reference range
• 30-100 units/L [SI units: 30-100 U/L]
Description
Enzyme amylase is generated in pancreas and salivary glands, which is released into blood on injury to pancreas (diseased or inflamed). It helps in assimilation of carbohydrates.

- **Increased:** Acute pancreatitis, pancreatic duct obstruction, alcohol ingestion, mumps, parotitis, renal disease, cholecystitis, peptic ulcers, intestinal obstruction, mesenteric thrombosis, postop abdominal surgery.
- **Decreased:** Liver damage, pancreatic destruction (pancreatitis, cystic fibrosis)

16.7 Angiotensin-converting Enzyme

Angiotensin-converting enzyme, serum
Reference range
<40 U/L [SI units: < 670 nkat/L]
Description
Important enzyme in the renin-angiotensin-aldosterone system and the kallikrein-kinin system. ACE's effects are based on direct vasoconstrictive effect of angiotensin II conversion from angiotensin I as well as increased catabolism of the vasodilatory bradykinins. ACE is found in the endothelial cells of the vascular system, particularly in the lungs and kidneys. Used as an indicator in the diagnosis of sarcoidosis.

Angiotensin-converting enzyme, serum (cont.)

Increased: Sarcoidosis (Boeck's disease), silicosis, asbestosis, tuberculosis, alcoholic liver disease, Gaucher's disease, kidney diseases, hyperparathyroidism, hyperthyroidism, diabetes mellitus

16.8   Anion Gap

Anion gap

Reference range

• 8-12 mEq/L [SI units: 8-12mmol/L]

Description

The anion gap is the difference between the major positive and negative ions in serum, plasma and urine.

Calculate: Anion gap = $(Na^+) - (HCO_3^- + Cl^-)$

- **Increased:** Lactic acidosis, high anion gap metabolic acidosis eg. DR. MAPLES (methanol, aspirin, paraldehyde/propylene glycol, lactic acid, ethylene glycol; ethanol ketoacidosis, starvation ketoacidosis)
- **Decreased:** Hypoalbuminemia, multiple myeloma, increased potassium, calcium, magnesium, lithium or bromide levels

16.9   Anti-nuclear Antibody (ANA)

Anti-nuclear antibody

Reference range

Negative ≤ 1:40

Description

The anti-nuclear antibody or ANA detects antibodies to all nuclear antigens present in serum by an indirect immunofluorescence assay. Since the test is non-specific, it may be positive in many autoimmune conditions and at low titers (1:40-1:80) in up to 20-25 % of normal persons. When positive at higher titers, autoimmune or connective tissue diseases are more likely, but more specific antibody testing is needed for better differentiation (shown below).

- **Positive:** Connective tissue disease - Systemic lupus erythematosus (anti-dsDNA; anti-Sm), drug-induced lupus (anti-histone), Sjögren's syndrome (anti-Ro/La), rheumatoid arthritis (rheumatoid factor; anti-CCP), scleroderma or systemic sclerosis (anti-Scl-70; anti-centromere), mixed connective tissue disease (anti-RNP), polymyositis or dermatomyositis (anti-PM-1; anti-Jo-1). Other conditions: Autoimmune hepatitis, primary biliary cirrhosis (anti-mitochondrial), chronic hepatitis C, ulcerative colitis, Crohn's disease, SBE
- **Negative:** Negative predictive value for lupus

16.10 Anti-neutrophil Cytoplasmic Antibody (ANCA)

Anti-neutrophil cytoplasmic antibody
Reference range
Positive: Confirm with anti-PR3 and anti-MPO titers
Description
ANCA tests for autoantibodies to antigens in neutrophil cytoplasm; c-ANCA staining diffusely in the cytoplasm and p-ANCA in a peri-nuclear pattern.

- **Positive:** c-ANCA, usually anti-proteinase 3 (PR3) - granulomatosis with polyangiitis (Wegener's), pauci-immune glomerulonephritis, Churg-Strauss syndrome, P-ANCA, usually anti-myeloperoxidase (MPO) - microscopic polyangiitis, pauci-immune necrotizing "renal-limited vasculitis" glomerulonephritis (may be positive in anti-GBM nephritis also), Churg-Strauss syndrome, drug-induced vasculitis, other connective tissue diseases, ulcerative colitis, Crohn's disease, autoimmune hepatitis, sclerosing cholangitis

16.11 Bilirubin

Reference range
• Total: 0.2-1.0 mg/dl [SI units: 3.42-17.1µmol/L]
• Direct: 0-0.3 mg/dl [SI units: 0-5.13 µmol/L]
• Indirect: 0.2-0.6 mg/dl [SI units: 3.42-10.26 µmol/L]
Description
Bile is produced by liver and which contains yellowish pigment bilirubin.

- **Increased total:** Hepatic damage (hepatitis, toxins, cirrhosis), biliary obstruction, hemolysis, fasting
- **Increased direct (conjugated):** Biliary obstruction / cholestasis, drug induced cholestasis.

16.12 BUN

Reference range
• 7-20 mg/dl [SI units: 2.5-7.14 mmol/L]
Description
The test evaluates the amount of urea nitrogen in the blood to evaluate kidney function. Urea is a by-product of protein breakdown produced by the liver.

- **Increased:** Acute kidney injury, renal failure, pre-renal azotemia (hypotension, septic" shock, volume depletion), postrenal (obstruction), GI bleeding, catabolic states, drugs (corticosteroids, amino acid infusions), high protein intake
- **Decreased:** Starvation, liver failure, pregnancy, infancy, overhydration

16.13 BUN:Cr Ratio

Reference range
• Between 10:1 and 20:1
Description
• **Increased:** Prenal failure, GI bleeding, catabolic states, postrenal obstruction, steroids and tetracycline
• **Decreased:** Hepatic insufficiency, rhabdomyolysis (creatinine rises more than BUN), malnutrition

16.14 Calcium

Calcium, serum
Reference range
Calcium, total, serum
• 8.2-10.2 mg/dL [SI units: 2.05-2.55 mmol/L]
Calcium, ionized, serum
• 4.60-5.08 mg/dL [SI units: 1.15-1.27 mmol/L]
Description
Calcium is essential for the proper contraction of the muscles and blood vessels and for the efficient conduction of impulses through the nervous system and in the secretion of hormones by the endocrine system. Bones and teeth act as the chief stores of calcium in the body along with blood and other tissues of the body.
• **Increased:** Malignancies- non-Hodgkin's lymphoma, multiple myeloma, breast and other cancers, primary hyperparathyroidism, tertiary hyperparathyroidism, hyperthyroidism, adrenal insufficiency, Paget's disease, 1, 25 dihydroxy vitamin D overproduction (tuberculosis, sarcoidosis, fungal diseases, berylliosis); Drugs: Hypervitaminosis of A or D, calcitriol, lithium, thiazides, theophylline toxicity, tamoxifen, milk-alkali syndrome
• **Decreased:** Hypoparathyroidism, insufficient vitamin D, hypomagnesemia, renal tubular acidosis, hypoalbuminemia, chronic renal failure (phosphate retention), acute pancreatitis, alcoholism

16.15 Calcitonin

Calcitonin
Reference range
3-26 pg/mL [SI units: 0.8-7.6 pmol/L]
Description
A hormone produced in the C cells of the thyroid gland that downregulates blood calcium, opposing the action of parathyroid hormone (PTH) and vitamin D.
• **Increased:** Malignant diseases- medullary thyroid cancer, lung cancer, insulinomas, VIPomas; non-malignant diseases- newborns, pregnancy, renal failure, Zollinger-Ellison syndrome (associated with men), pernicious anemia

16.16 Chloride

Chloride, serum
Reference range
• 98-108 mEq/L [SI units: 98-108 mmol/L]
Description
Chloride is the major anion maintaining the electrical and acid base balance of the body and regulating the reabsorption and maintenance of sodium and fluids in the body.
• **Increased:** Metabolic acidosis (non-anion gap), respiratory alkalosis (compensated), renal tubular acidosis
• **Decreased:** Addison's disease, burns, congestive heart failure, dehydration, excessive sweating, metabolic alkalosis, respiratory acidosis (compensated), syndrome of inappropriate diuretic hormone (SIADH) secretion and other hyponatremic states.
Chloride, urine
Reference range
• 110-250 mEq/day [SI units: 110-250 mmol/day]
• Varies with diet
Description
Same as above for chloride.
• **Increased:** Dehydration, starvation, Addison disease, increased salt intake
• **Decreased:** Cushing syndrome, Conn syndrome, congestive heart failure, malabsorption syndrome, diarrhea, decreased salt intake

16.17 Complement (C3, C4)

Serum Complement (C3, C4)
Reference range
C3: 90-180 mg/dL [SI units: 0.9-1.8 g/L] C4: 10-40 mg/dL [SI units: 0.1-0.4 g/L]
Description
The complement system is part of the body's immune and inflammatory response and testing is used to evaluate immune and autoimmune disorders. While normal in-creases occur in infectious illnesses, complement is most often measured to detect autoimmune conditions that lower serum complement levels by binding and/or consumption of complement components. • **Increased:** Acute response to infection or injury • **Decreased:** Lupus, Sjögren's syndrome, cryoglobulinemia, immune complex and membranoproliferative glomerulonephritis, serum sickness, hemolysis, and in-heri-ted complement disorders

16.18 Creatinine Clearance

Reference range
Normal creatinine production and excretion is: • Males: 15-20 mg/Kg/24h • Females: 10-15 mg/Kg/24h Normal creatinine clearance is: • Male: 97-137 mL/min [SI units: 1.6-2.2 mL/s] • Female: 88-128 mL/min [SI units: 1.4-2.1 mL/s]
Description
The creatinine clearance test helps detect and diagnose kidney dysfunction and disorders of renal perfusion. It is a measure of the efficiency of the filtration process of the kidneys, evaluated by comparing the level of creatinine excreted in the urine to the creatinine levels in the blood. Creatinine clearance = U_{Cr} (in mg/dL) x U_{Vol} (in ml/min)/S_{Cr} (in mg/dL) • **Increased:** High protein intake, early diabetes mellitus, burns, CO poisioning, hypothyroidism, pregnancy. • **Decreased:** Acute and chronic kidney injury or renal failure, congestive heart failure, dehydration.

16.19 Creatinine

Creatinine, serum
Reference range
• Male: 0.7-1.2 mg/dL [SI units: 61.8-106 µmol/L]
• Female: 0.6-1.1 mg/dL [SI units: 53-97 µmol/L]
Description
Creatinine is a breakdown product of muscle metabolism, it is filtered out of the blood by kidneys. The test is used to measure functioning of kidneys. If kidney function is altered then creatinine levels rise in blood.
• **Increased:** Acute or chronic renal failure, urinary tract obstruction, drugs which decrease kidney function or tubular creatinine secretion (eg, trimethoprim), body building or creatine intake
• **Decreased:** Muscle atrophy, protein starvation, liver disease, pregnancy

16.20 Cystatin C

Cystatin C, serum
Reference range
• Male: 0.56-0.98 mg/L
• Female: 0.52-0.90 mg/L
Description
Cystatin C is a 120 amino acid, basic protein secreted by all nucleated cells and removed by glomerular filtration. It can be used to estimate GFR (see CKD chapter →205) with less effect of age, race and muscle mass than creatinine, but it is affected by body composition, cancer and various other conditions.
• **Increased:** Acute or chronic renal failure, HIV, increased BMI, high C-reactive protein, hyperthyroidism, corticosteroid use, and other disorders
• **Decreased:** Atherosclerotic vascular disease, cyclosporine Rx

16.21 Fractional Excretion of Sodium (FENa %)

Reference range
• <1 %
Description
FENa is the quantity (percentage) of sodium excreted in the urine compared to the amount filtered by the kidney and is used as a test to distinguish prerenal from renal causes of kidney injury/failure.
FeNa = Na+ excreted/Na+ filtered = $(U_{Na} \times S_{Cr} \times 100)/(S_{Na} \times U_{Cr})$

Fractional Excretion of Sodium (cont.)
• **Increased:** Acute tubular necrosis (>1%, often >3%)
• **Decreased:** Prerenal azotemia (<1%)

16.22 Ferritin

Ferritin, serum
Reference range
15-200 ng/mL [SI units: 33-450 pmol/L]
Description
Ferritin is a protein that stores iron. The amount of ferritin gives an indication of the amount of iron stored in blood.
• **Increased:** Hemochromatosis and iron overload, inflammation, liver disease, chronic infection, autoimmune disorders, hemolytic anemia, sideroblastic anemia
• **Decreased:** Iron deficiency.

16.23 GFR

GFR, measured and estimated (eGFR)
Reference range
Measured GFR in young adults (decreasing with age):
• Male: 115-145 ml/min/1.73m^2
• Female: 105-140 mL/min/m^2
• Estimated eGFR: >60 mL/min/1.73m^2
Description
Glomerular filtration rate (GFR) test measures functioning of kidney and progression of CKD. Glomerular filtration is the process by which the kidneys filter the blood, removing excess wastes and fluids. GFR can be measured directly, as with inulin or iothalamate, or estimated from serum creatinine as below. $eGFR = 141 \times \min(Scr/\kappa, 1)^\alpha \times \max(Scr/\kappa, 1)^{-1.209} \times 0.993^{Age} \times 1.018$ [if female] $\times 1.159$ [if black], where Scr is serum creatinine (mg/dL), κ is 0.7 for females and 0.9 for males, α is −0.329 for females and −0.411 for males, min indicates the minimum of Scr/κ or 1, and max indicates the maximum of Scr/κ or 1 with a calculator at website: http://www.kidney.org/professionals/kdoqi/gfr.cfm
• **Increased:** Pregnancy, early diabetes
• **Decreased:** Acute or chronic kidney disease, volume depletion, hypotension, CHF

16.24 Glucose

Glucose, blood
Reference range
• Fasting blood glucose: 70-100 mg/dL [SI units: 3.9-5.5 mmol/L] • Random blood glucose: below 125 mg/dL [SI units: 6.88 mmol/L] • Impaired fasting glucose: 100-125 mg/dL [SI units: 5.5-6.88 mmol/L]
Description
Measuring glucose levels in the blood gives an indication of carbohydrate metabolism and balance of glycogen breakdown, gluconeogenesis, and glucose uptake mediated largely by insulin.
• **Increased:** Acromegaly, acute stress (response to trauma, heart attack, and stroke for instance), chronic kidney failure, Cushing syndrome, diabetes mellitus, excessive food intake, hyperthyroidism, pancreatic cancer, pancreatitis • **Decreased:** Adrenal insufficiency, drinking excessive alcohol, severe liver disease, hypopituitarism, hypothyroidism, insulin overdose, insulinomas, starvation.

Glucose, urine
Reference range
• Negative
Description
The glucose test is used in measuring the glucose levels in urine. Urinary excretion of glucose is called glycosuria or glucosuria.
• **Increased:** Diabetes mellitus, gestational diabetes, Acromegaly, estrogens and chloral hydrate, corticosteroids.

16.25 HCO_3^-

HCO_3^-, serum (also called bicarbonate or total CO_2)
Reference range
• Arterial: 21-27 mEq/L [SI units: 21-27 mmol/L] • Venous: 22-29 mEq/L [SI units: 22-29 mmol/L]
Description
Bicarbonate is a buffer that maintains the pH of blood from getting too acidic or too basic.
• **Increased:** Severe vomiting, pulmonary insufficiency, Cushing syndrome, hyperaldosteronism, metabolic alkalosis. • **Decreased:** Addison's disease, chronic diarrhea, diabetic ketoacidosis, metabolic acidosis, kidney disease, ethylene glycol or methanol poisoning

16.26 Hemoglobin (Hb)

Hemoglobin (Hb)

Reference range
- Male: 13.8-17.2 gm/dL [SI units: 138-172 g/L]
- Female: 12.1-15.1 gm/dL [SI units: 121-151 g/L]

Description

Oxygen-carrying pigment and major protein in erythrocytes. Hemoglobin forms an unstable, reversible bond with oxygen. Oxyhemoglobin (oxygenated state) transports oxygen from the lungs to the tissues where it releases its oxygen and converts to deoxyhemoglobin (deoxygenated state).

Increased: Polycythemia, volume depletion, hypoxia
Decreased: Anemia (hemorrhagic, hemolytic, or failure of RBC production)

16.27 Hematocrit

Hematocrit, whole blood

Reference range
- Male: 40-52%
- Female: 36-48%

Description

Packed cell volume (PCV, Hct): Proportion of the blood by volume that consists of RBCs, expressed as a percentage.

- **Increased:** Polycythemia, volume depletion, hypoxia
- **Decreased:** Anemia (hemorrhagic, hemolytic, or failure of RBC production)

16.28 Iron

Iron, serum

Reference range
- Male: 65-175 µg/dl [11.6-31.3 µmol/L]
- Female: 50-170 µg/dl [9.0-30.4 µmol/L]

Description

The total iron content of the body is approx. 38 mg/kg in women and 50 mg/kg in men. The iron stores in the body are: erythrocytes: approx. 3000 mg; myoglobin: approx. 120 mg; cytochromes: approx. 3-8 mg; liver/spleen: approx. 300- 800 mg. Daily turnover through synthesis and conversion of hemoglobin is 25 mg. Uptake occurs mainly through uptake of bivalent iron in the small intestine. Considerable iron loss is possible through menstruation, hemodialysis, and pregnancy.

Iron, serum (cont.)

- **Increased:** Hemochromatosis, hemolytic anemia, sideroblastic anemia, lead poisoning, liver disease
- **Decreased:** Iron deficiency, chronic illness, poor diet, intestinal disease (problems with absorption), hemodialysis, parasitic diseases

16.29 Ketones

Ketones, urine

Reference range

- Negative
- When ketones are present in the urine, the results are usually listed as small, moderate, or large with these corresponding values:
  - Small: <20 mg/dL
  - Moderate: 30 - 40 mg/dL
  - Large: > 80 mg/dL

Description

Ketones are made in excess when fat is metabolized preferentially more than carbohydrates to supply energy.

- **Increased:** Anorexia, fasting, diabetic ketoacidosis, high fat or low carbohydrate diets, starvation, vomiting over a long period of time, alcoholism, acute or severe illness, burns, fever

16.30 Lactate

Lactate, plasma

Reference range

5.0-18 mg/dL [SI units: 0.6-2.0 mmol/L]

Description

Lactic acid is produced from the metabolism of glucose when pyruvic acid is converted to lactic acid. Since the H^+ ion will be picked up by the body's buffers, excess lactate will reduce the serum bicarbonate, causing an anion gap metabolic acidosis. Note that lactate measurement only detects L-lactate, not D-lactic acidosis from bacterial metabolism in short bowel syndromes.

- **Increased** (> 4.0 mmol/L): Tissue ischemia (shock, sepsis), drugs (metformin, zidovudine, stavudine, didanosine), alcoholism, malignancy

16.31 Magnesium

Magnesium, serum
Reference range
1.5-2.6 mEq/L [SI units: 0.62-1.07 mmol/L]
Description
Distribution within the body has some similarity to potassium, with approx. 1% (mainly in ionized form) in the serum, approx. 40% in the skeletal muscles and approx. 60% in bones. Important for many enzymes, including the activation of Na^+ K^+ ATPase (significant for cardiac dysrhythmias), adenylate cyclase, pyruvate dehydrogenase, calcium ATPase and others.
• **Increased:** Renal insufficiency, uncontrolled diabetes mellitus, Addison's disease, hypothyroidism, drugs - magnesium-containing antacids or enema salts
• **Decreased:** Malabsorption syndromes, alcoholism, chronic inflammatory bowel diseases, sprue, chronic renal disease, diabetic acidosis, diuretics, nephrotoxic drugs

16.32 Osmolality

Osmolality, plasma (pOSM)
Reference range
• 275-295 mOsm/kg [SI units: 275-295 mmol/kg]
Description
The test is used for measuring blood osmolality, primarily proportional to sodium and its accompanying anion, glucose and urea.
• **Increased:** Dehydration, hyperglycemia, hypernatremia, kidney failure with azotemia, mannitol therapy, alcohol, ethylene glycol or methanol toxicity
• **Decreased:** Excess hydration, hyponatremia, inappropriate ADH secretion

Osmolality, urine (uOSM)
Reference range
• 50 - 1200 mOsm/kg [SI units: 50-1200 mmol/kg]
Description
The testing of urine osmolality is important in the diagnosis of conditions that cause an increased urinary volume. Urine osmolality should be tested in renal concentration defects, diabetes insipidus, osmotic diuresis and water diuresis. The human antidiuretic hormone (ADH) is arginine-vasopressin (AVP) whose release is regulated by an increase in plasma osmolality or by a reduction in the intravascular volume (extracellular volume). AVP causes a reduction (antidiuresis) of water excretion. When plasma osmolality is <280 mosmol/kg H_2O, AVP release should be low, when osmolality increases to >300 mosmol/kg H_2O, AVP release is increased with concentrated urine.
• **Increased:** Congestive heart failure, hypernatremia, inappropriate ADH secretion, liver damage, shock
• **Decreased:** Diabetes insipidus, excess fluid intake, hypercalcemia, hypokalemia, kidney tubular damage

16.33 Parathyroid Hormone (PTH)

Parathyroid Hormone
Reference range
• 10 - 65 picograms per milliliter (pg/mL) [SI units: 10-65 ng/L]
Description
Peptide hormone formed in the parathyroid glands whose function is to raise the serum calcium by causing bone resorption and calcium reabsorption by the renal tubules and to lower serum phosphate by inhibiting phosphate reabsorption by the renal tubules.
• **Increased:** Osteitis fibrosa, extraskeletal calcification, calciphylaxis, chronic kidney disease, hypersecretion or adenoma of the parathyroid glands
• **Decreased:** Osteomalacia, adynamic/aplastic bone lesions, low levels of magnesium in the blood, radiation to the parathyroid glands, sarcoidosis, vitamin D intoxication

16.34 pH

Reference range
- Arterial: 7.36–7.44
- Venous: 7.33–7.43

Description

Blood gas analysis is done to determine the pH. Most commonly, gas analysis is done on arterial blood (ABG) to categorically determine the level of oxygenation and to assess whether disturbances in the pH and buffering system of arterial blood are due to respiratory or metabolic causes. Ideally, the pH of the blood should be maintained at 7.4 and which is kept constant by buffers dissolved in the blood.

- **Increased:** Metabolic alkalosis (eg, vomiting, diuretics), respiratory alkalosis
- **Decreased:** Metabolic acidosis, non-anion gap (DR. DOOFUS-diarrhea, RTA, drugs as acetazolamide, topiramate, ifosfamide, or tenofovir, obstructive uropathy, other as recovery from hyperventilation, fistulous ileal bladder, uremia, sniffing glue) or high anion gap (DR. MAPLES - diabetic ketoacidosis, renal failure, methanol, aspirin, paraldehyde or propylene glycol, lactic acid, ethylene glycol or ethanol ketoacidosis, starvation ketoacidosis), respiratory acidosis.

16.35 pO_2

Reference range
- Arterial: 80–100 mmHg [SI units: 10.6-13.3 kPa]
- Venous: 37–47 mmHg [SI units: 5-6.3 kPa]

Description

It measures the partial pressures of oxygen in the blood. An ABG analysis evaluates how effectively the lungs are delivering oxygen to the blood.

- **Increased:** Oxygen assistance by O2 mask or nasal cannula
- **Decreased:** COPD, pneumonia, hypoventilation or increased alveolar-arterial gradient

16.36 pCO_2

Reference range
- Arterial: 35–45 mmHg [SI units: 4.7-5.9 kPa]
- Venous: 36–48 mmHg [SI units: 4.7-6.4 kPa]

Description

It measures the partial pressures of carbon dioxide in the blood. An ABG analysis evaluates how effectively the lungs are eliminating carbon dioxide.

pCO$_2$ (cont.)
• **Increased:** Respiratory acidosis, hypoventilation, metabolic alkalosis (compensation)
• **Decreased:** Respiratory alkalosis, hyperventilation, sepsis, liver disease, pregnancy, salicylate toxicity, metabolic acidosis (compensation)

16.37 Phosphorus

Phosphorus, serum
Reference range
• 2.7–4.5 mg/dl [SI units: 0.87–1.45mmol/L]
Description
85% of phosphate is contained in bones and teeth, 14% in body cells and 1% in the extracellular space. Energy-rich phosphates (ATP) supply energy for metabolic reactions.
• **Increased:** Acute and chronic renal failure, acidosis (lactic acidosis, diabetic ketoacidosis), phosphate administration, phosphate-containing laxatives, tumor lysis syndrome, osteolytic metastases, vitamin D overdose, hypoparathyroidism, pseudohypoparathyroidism, hyperthyroidism
• **Decreased:** Primary hyperparathyroidism, renal tubular defects, postrenal transplantation, ECF volume expansion, hyperaldosteronism, hypokalemia, hypercalcemia, hypomagnesemia, Cushing's syndrome, mesenchymoma, neurofibroma, vomiting, diarrhea, malabsorption, drugs: steroid therapy, oral contraceptives, estrogens, diuretics

16.38 Potassium

Potassium, serum
Reference range
• 3.5 - 5.1 mEq/L [SI units: 3.5 - 5.1 mmol/L]
Description
Potassium is closely regulated between the intracellular and extracellular fluid compartments, most of the body stores in muscle and bone. The potassium electrical potential across cardiac cell membranes is important to heart function so that severe hyperkalemia or hypokalemia need immediate attention and treatment.
• **Decreased:** Diarrhea, vomiting, severe sweating, Cushing syndrome, hyperaldosteronism, Bartter or Gitelman syndrome, Fanconi syndrome, diuretics, antibiotics-amphotericin, high dose penicillin, gentamicin
• **Increased:** Addison's disease, acute or chronic kidney failure, ACE inhibitors, ARBs, beta-blockers, K-sparing diuretics (spironolactone, eplerenone, amiloride, triamterene), trimethoprim

16.39 Protein/creatinine Ratio

Protein/creatinine ratio, urine

Reference range

- Normal: <0.2
- Moderate proteinuria: 0.3-2.9
- Nephrotic range proteinuria: >3.0

Description

Protein/creatinine ratio measures all urinary proteins, not just albumin, so immune globulins and polypeptides are included. The test is helpful to assess severity and to follow proteinuric kidney diseases.

- **Positive:** Proteinuric glomerular diseases, renal tubular proteinuria, multiple myeloma and other dysglobulinemias

16.40 SaO$_2$

Oxygen Saturation (hemoglobin)

Reference range

- Arterial: >95%
- Venous: 60–85%

Description

Oxygen saturation measures how much of the hemoglobin in the red blood cells is carrying oxygen.

- **Increased:** Oxygen assistance by O2 mask or nasal cannula
- **Decreased:** COPD, pneumonia, hypoventilation or increased alveolar-arterial gradient

16.41 Sodium

Sodium, serum

Reference range

- 135 to 145 mEq/L [135 to 145 mmol/L]

Description

Sodium constitutes 90%-95% of all cations in the blood plasma and interstitial fluid and it thus determines most of the osmolality and volume of the extracellular fluid.

Sodium, serum (cont.)

- **Decreased:** Addison's disease, glucocorticoid deffigiency, severe heart failure, cirrhosis, diarrhea, diuretics, burns, pancreatitis, acute hyperglycemia, severe lipemia or hyperglobulinemia may cause pseudohyponatremia
- **Increased:** Dehydration, Cushing syndrome, diabetes insipidus, hyperaldosteronism, osmotic diuresis, prolonged glucosuria.

Sodium, urine

Reference range

- 40-220 mEq/day (Varies with dietary intake)

Description

It measures the amount of sodium excreted in urine during 24 hours. Sodium maintains water and electrolyte balance of body.

- **Decreased:** Volume depletion, congestive heart failure, liver disease, nephrotic syndrome, low salt intake
- **Increased:** Diuretic use, Addison's disease, high salt intake

16.42 Specific Gravity

Specific gravity, urine

Reference range

- 1.003 to 1.030

Description

Test measures the density of urine and is usually proportional to the osmolality or concentration of the urine. However, dense substances, such as radiocontrast or glucose, increase density and specific gravity much more than osmolality.

- **Increased:** Dehydration, diarrhea, glucosuria, heart failure, renal arterial stenosis, shock, syndrome of inappropriate antidiuretic hormone secretion (SIADH)
- **Decreased:** Excessive fluid intake, diabetes insipidus, hypercalcemia, hypokalemia, kidney tubular damage

16.43 Total Iron Binding Capacity (TIBC)

Reference range
• 250–425 µg/dl [SI units: 44.8–76.1 µmol/L]

Description
Total iron-binding capacity (TIBC) is most frequently used to evaluate iron deficiency or iron overload. It is used along with a serum iron test to calculate the transferrin saturation to determine how much iron is being carried in the blood. • **Increased:** Iron deficiency anemia, pregnancy, use of oral contraceptives. • **Decreased:** Cirrhosis, hemolytic anemia, hypoproteinemia, inflammation, liver disease, malnutrition, pernicious anemia, sickle cell anemia, nephrotic syndrome.

16.44 Transferrin Saturation

Reference range
• Males: 15–50% • Females: 12–45%

Description
Transferrin is capable of associating reversibly with iron and acting as an iron trans-porting protein. Transferrin saturation (%) = 100 x serum iron (µg/dl) / TIBC (µg/dl) is only diagnostically relevant in conjunction with iron and ferritin levels. • **Increased:** Iron overload or poisoning, hemochromatosis, hemolytic anemia, sideroblastic anemia, starvation, nephrotic syndrome, cirrhosis • **Decreased:** Iron deficiency anemia, chronic infection, chronic inflammation, uremia, third trimester of pregnancy

16.45 Uric Acid

Uric acid, serum
Reference range
• Male: 3.4–7.5 mg/dL [SI units 202–446 µmol/L] • Female: 2.4–6.0 mg/dL [SI units 143–357 µmol/L]

Description
Uric acid is produced from the break-down of purines, requiring the enzyme xan-thine oxidase, mainly located in the liver and small intestine. Uric acid elimination occurs about 80 % in the kidney and about 20% in the intestines. Complications of hyperuricemia are acute gouty arthritis, chronic soft tissue- and/or bone tophi, nephrolithiasis, and acute uric acid nephropathy. • **Increased:** Gout, multiple myeloma, metastatic cancer, leukemia, diet high in purines, diuretics, kidney insufficiency • **Decreased:** Allopurinol, pregnancy, probenicid

17 Appendix

17.1 List of Abbreviations

↑	Increased or elevated
↓	Decreased or depressed
⇒	Leads to
α	Alpha
β	Beta
Ca^{++}	Calcium ion
Cl^-	Chloride ion
H^+	Hydrogen ion
iCa^{++}	Ionized calcium
K^+	Potassium ion
HCO_3^-	Bicarbonate
pCO_2	Carbon dioxide partial pressure
pH	Negative log of the hydrogen ion concentration
pKa	Negative log of the acid dissociation constant
A	Surface area
Ab	Antibody
ABG	Arterial blood gases
ABx	Antibiotic treatment
ACE	Angiotensin-converting enzyme
ACEI	Angiotensin-converting enzyme inhibitor
ACTH	Adrenocorticotropic hormone
ACR	Albumin to creatinine ratio
ADH	Anti diuretic hormone
ADPKD	Autosomal dominant polycystic kidney disease

AFP	Alpha fetoprotein
AG	Anion gap
AIDS	Acquired immune deficiency syndrome
AIHA	Autoimmune hemolytic anemia
AIN	Acute interstitial nephritis
AKI	Acute kidney injury
AKIN	Acute kidney injury network
ALG	Anti-lymphocyte globulin
ALLHAT	The Antihypertensive and Lipid-Lowering Treatment to Prevent Heart Attack Trial
ANA	Antinuclear antibody
ANCA	Antineutrophil cytoplasmic autoantibody
ANP	Atrial natriuretic peptide
APC	Antigen-presenting cells
APD	Automated peritoneal dialysis
ARB	Angiotensin receptor blocker
ARF	Acute renal failure
ASA	Aspirin (acetylsalicylic acid)
ATN	Acute tubular necrosis
ATGAM	Anti-lymphocyte immune globulin
AV	Arteriovenous
AVF	Arterio-venous fistula
AVG	Arterio-venous graft
BB	Beta-blocker
BMI	Body mass index

BNP	Brain natriuretic peptide	COPD	Chronic obstructive pulmonary disease
BSA	Body surface area	COX-1 & 2	Cyclooxygenase-1 & 2
BUN	Blood urea nitrogen	C_{Cr}/CrCl	Creatinine clearance
BW	Body weight	Cr	Creatinine
Ca	Calcium	CRP	C-reactive protein
CaCO3	Calcium carbonate	CRRT	Continuous renal replacement therapy
cAMP	Cyclic adenosine monophosphate	CT	Computed tomography
CAN	Chronic allograft nephropathy	CVA	Costovertebral angle
CAPD	Continuous ambulatory peritoneal dialysis	CVC	Central venous catheter
CAVH	Continuous arterio-venous hemofiltration	CVVH	Continuous veno-venous hemofiltration
CBC	Complete blood count	CVVHD	Continuous veno-venous hemodiafiltration
CCB	Calcium channel blocker	CXR	Chest X-ray
CCPD	Continuous cycling peritoneal dialysis	D	Dialysate
CFPD	Continuous flow peritoneal dialysis	DDAVP	Desmopressin (1-deamino-8-D-arginine vasopressin)
CHF	Congestive heart failure	DI	Diabetes insipidus
CIN	Chronic interstitial nephritis	DIC	Disseminated intravascular coagulation
CKD	Chronic kidney disease	DGF	Delayed graft function
CKD-EPI	Chronic kidney disease epidemiology collaboration (CKD-EPI) expression	dL	Deciliter
Cl	Chloride	DM	Diabetes mellitus
CLIA	Clinical laboratory improvement amendments	DTPA	Diethylenetriaminepentacetic acid
CLL	Chronic lymphocytic leukemia	EBV	Epstein–barr virus
CMV	Cytomegalovirus	ECF	Extracellular fluid
CNI	Calcineurin inhibitors	ECG	Electrocardiography
CNS	Central nervous system	EDTA	Ethylenediaminetetraacetic Acid
CO	Carbon monoxide	EEG	Electroencephalography

ELISA	Enzyme-linked immunosorbent assay
EM	Electron microscopy
EPO	Erythropoietin
ER	Energy requirement
ESR	Erythrocyte sedimentation rate
ESRD or ESKD	End-stage renal disease or end-stage kidney disease
ESWL	Extracorporeal shock wave lithotripsy
FCXM	Flow cytometric crossmatch
FE	Fractional excretion
FENa	Fractional excretion of sodium
FGF 23	Fibroblast growth factor 23
FSGS	Focal segmental glomerular sclerosis
GBM	Glomerular basement membrane
GF	Growth factor
GFR	Glomerular filtration rate
GI	Gastrointestinal
gm	Gram
GN	Glomerulonephritis
GST	Glutathione S-transferase
HAART	Highly active antiretroviral therapy
Hb	Hemoglobin
HbA1c	Hemoglobin A1c (glycosylated hemoglobin)
hCG	Human chorionic gonadotropin
HCV	Hepatitis C virus

HCTZ	Hydrochlorothiazide
HD	Hemodialysis
HELLP (syndrome)	H – hemolysis (the breakdown of red blood cells); EL - elevated liver enzymes; LP - low platelet count
HLA	Human leukocyte antigen
H_2O	Water
HIV	Human immunodeficiency virus
HRCT	High-resolution chest computed tomography
HSP	Henoch-Schönlein Purpura
HSV	Herpes simplex virus
HTN	Hypertension
HUS	Hemolytic uremic syndrome
Hx & Px	History & physical exam
IBW	Ideal body weight
ICAM	Intercellular adhesion molecule
ICF	Intracellular fluid
IF	Immunofluorescent microscopy
IGF	Insulin-like growth factor
I & O	Intake & output
IL	Interleukin
IM	Intramuscular
INR	International normalized ratio (of prothrombin time)
IPD	Intermittent peritoneal dialysis
ISF	Interstitial fluid
IV	Intravascular

IVC	Inferior vena cava
IVF	Intravascular fluid
IVP	Intravenous pyelography
JNC	The Joint National Committee
JVD	Jugular venous distension
K	Potassium
KFT	Kidney function test
kg/Kg	Kilogram
Ko	Mass transfer coefficient
KDIGO	Kidney disease: Improving global outcomes
KIM-1	Kidney injury molecule-1
KUB	Kidney, ureter, and bladder
L	Liter/Liters
LAM	Lymphangioleiomyomatosis
L-FABP	Liver fatty-acid binding protein
LM	Light microscopy
LVH	Left ventricular hypertrophy
MCD	Minimal change disease
MCV	Mean corpuscular volume
MDRD	Modification of diet in renal disease (study)
mEq	Milliequivalents
mg	Milligram
MGUS	Monoclonal gammopathy of undetermined significance
MHC	Major histocompatibility complex
MMF	Mycophenolate mofetil
MPA	Mycophenolic acid
MPGN	Membranoproliferative glomerulonephritis

MRA	Magnetic resonance angiography
MRI	Magnetic resonance imaging
MRSA	Methicillin-resistant Staphylococcus aureus
MSSA	Methicillin susceptible Staphylococcus aureus
mTOR	The mammalian target of rapamycin
Na	Sodium
NaCl	Sodium chloride
$NaHCO_3$	Sodium bicarbonate
NAC	N-acetylcysteine
NAG	N-acetyl-betaglucosaminidase
NGAL	Neutrophil gelatinase-associated lipocalin
NIPD	Nocturnal intermittent peritoneal dialysis
NO	Nitric oxide
NPHP	Nephronophthisis
NS	Normal saline
NSAIDS	Non-steroidal anti-inflammatory drugs
Osm	Osmolality
P	Plasma
PBS	Peripheral blood smear
PAPP-A	Pregnancy-associated plasma protein
PCKD	Polycystic kidney disease
PCN	Penicillin
PCR	Protein to creatinine ratio
PD	Peritoneal dialysis

310 17 Appendix

PET	Peritoneal equilibration test
PFT	Pulmonary function test
PGE1/PGE2	Prostaglandin E1/E2
PGI2	Prostacyclin
PIGN	Postinfectious glomerulonephritis
PKD	Polycystic kidney disease
POD	Post operative day
PRA	Panel reactive antibodies
PSGN	Poststreptococcal glomerulonephritis
PTH	Parathyroid hormone, parathormone or parathyrin
PTHrP	Parathyroid hormone-related protein
PTLD	Post-transplant lymphoproliferative disorder
PTT	Partial thromboplastin time
RAS	Renal artery stenosis
RBC	Red blood cell
RHC	Right-sided heart catheterization
RNA	Ribonucleic acid
RPGN	Rapidly progressive glomerulonephritis
RRT	Renal replacement therapy
RTA	Renal tubular acidosis
Rx	Treatment or prescription
SaO2	Oxygen saturation
SC	Subcutaneous

SCr or S_{Cr}	Serum creatinine
SG	Specific gravity
SIADH	Syndrome of inappropriate antidiuretic hormone secretion
SLE	Systemic lupus erythematosus
S_{Osm}	Serum osmolality
SSc	Systemic sclerosis/scleroderma
STD	Sexually transmitted diseases
TB	Tuberculosis
TBW	Total body water
TFT	Thyroid function tests
TGF	Transforming growth factor
TIBC	Total iron binding capacity
TINU	Tubulointerstitial nephritis-uveitis syndrome
TMA	Thrombotic microangiopathy
TNF	Tumor necrosis factor
tPA	Tissue plasminogen activator
TPD	Tidal peritoneal dialysis
TRH	Thyrotropin-releasing hormone
TSAT	Transferrin saturation
TTKG	Transtubular potassium gradient
TTP	Thrombotic thrombocytopenic purpura
U	Units
UA	Urinalysis
U_{Cl}	Chloride - urine
U_K	Potassium - urine
U_{Na}	Sodium - urine

UO	Urine output
UPEP & SPEP	Urine & serum protein electro-phoresis
URR	Urea reduction ratio
US	Ultrasound
UTI	Urinary tract infection
VDRL	The Venereal Disease Research Laboratory test
V/Q scan	Ventilation/perfusion scan
VRE	Vancomycin-resistant entero-cocci
vWF	von Willebrand factor
WBC's	White blood cells
WHO	World Health Organization
wk(s)	week(s)

17.2   Useful Addresses/websites

American Society of Nephrology
www.asn-online.org/

National Kidney Foundation (NKF)
http://www.kidney.org/

NKF eGFR Calculator
http://www.kidney.org/professionals/kdoqi/gfr.cfm

Journal of the American Society of Nephrology
jasn.asnjournals.org/

American Society of Transplantation (AST)
www.a-s-t.org/

American Association of Kidney Patients
www.aakp.org/

American Nephrology Nurses' Association
www.annanurse.org/

International Society of Nephrology (ISN) Gateway - The ISN Website
www.theisn.org/

KDOQI Guidelines
www.kidney.org/professionals/kdoqi/

Kidney Disease: Improving Global Outcomes (KDIGO) Guidelines
http://www.kdigo.org/

American Journal of Kidney Diseases
www.ajkd.org/

American Journal of Nephrology
http://www.karger.com/Journal/Home/223979

Peritoneal Dialysis International
www.pdiconnect.com/

International Society for Peritoneal Dialysis
http://ispd.org/

Renal Physicians Association
www.renalmd.org/

Renal Pathology Society
www.renalpathsoc.org/

Numerics

A

B

Trade name = **bold**   *Drug name = italic*

Trade name = bold   Drug name = italic

Trade name = **bold**   Drug name = *italic*

Notes